THINK SMART

AND

LIVE LONG

A REVIEW OF HEALTH CARE

By

Morris "J" Llewellyn

ISBN: 1-4033-4762-X (e-book)
ISBN: 1-4033-4763-8 (Paperback)
ISBN: 1-4033-4764-6 (Hardcover)
ISBN: 1-4033-4765-4 (RocketBook)

This book is printed on acid free paper.

1stBooks – rev. 10/30/02

DISCLAIMER

The essence of this message is repeated a number of times in the pages of this book because I want to make several points very clear.

The information in this book comes from personal experience and study. I offer it to others who want to benefit by what I know to be true. Although I may be critical of the medical establishment at times, I support and respect the average medical doctor who operates from day to day with the knowledge he has been given and I recognize his valiant effort to heal his patients and help his fellow man.

This book is informational only and is not intended to be used for diagnosis or treatment of any health disorder.

I encourage others to do as I have done: Use the effective diagnostic and health treatments made available by the establishment. Make sure your health care professional is properly trained and duly licensed. Please note that there are many approaches to health care. I urge the use of wisdom and caution in the selection of appropriate medical services.

The author is not a medical doctor and does not offer any of this information as medical advise. Therefore, neither he nor the publisher take responsibility for the way information in this book is used.

TABLE OF CONTENTS

CREDITS

If I have reached my audience, if my message is understandable and if the writing mechanics are adequate, all the credit belongs to a woman who is helpful and tolerant beyond measure. That would be my wife Marlene.

INTRODUCTION

The introduction to this book is essential to the reader being able to understand my purpose, my intense interest in health issues, and the reasons why this book was written.

I was born in a small Utah town in 1927. These were difficult years of the great depression. Doctors, midwives, and other health practitioners of the times were very willing to travel in open country making house calls. It was common back then for health practitioners to vary greatly in their skills and backgrounds. From that time to this I have had an interest in how healing takes place and what roles are played by the patient, the health practitioner, and the unknown forces of the universe. I still see a significant influence by all of these elements in the healing process.

The advancement of science has (in my mind) only increased the evidence that there are many influences in the healing process and that today we are faced with an even greater body of the unknown. Each time we discover a new dimension of understanding we open up a vast universe of unknowns. The work in genetic research and DNA exemplifies this principle.

This book is a partial personal history which reveals a great deal of information about health practices. It reflects what I have learned about staying healthy, getting sick, reversing the disease process and regaining good health.

This book is not intended to be a technical reference. Therefore, there is no index. A table of contents serves as an outline of subject material. For the benefit of serious students wishing to pursue these subjects in greater detail, I recommend using included references which appear in the text and at the end of some chapters.

The reason for an unusual format and a lot of brevity in a field that is very detailed is the need for simplicity and understanding.

Our greatest inability to solve a problem often rests with the inability to properly identify the problem. A number of extremely difficult situations exist in our health care systems. These situations need to be understood before we can realize solutions. Research and government are especially burdened by a disorder called "analysis paralysis". Detailed information and excessive procedures overwhelm effective communication.

In the medical field doctors and patients are both victimized. Pressures for greater profits are probably the number one cause. A stream of new medicines improperly introduced into medical practice are overwhelming doctors and endangering patients. Efforts external to medical practice are injected into the system which endanger patients and breakdown the doctor/patient relationship. One of the main problems is the extensive use of HMO's.

Yesterdays science has become today's lie. Profit opportunities bury truth for the purpose of perpetuating profit whether it be in government, business, or medical research.

The world is in political, social, religious, economic, and scientific turmoil. What is true? What is false? Much of the time it is hard to tell. This book only deals with the health care issue. I have tried to relate what I have done on my own. I hope I have shed some light on what we all can do about these issues. I implore you to exercise your rights and do what you can for yourself. If you do, it will ultimately benefit us all.

Morris J. Llewellyn
Author

Part I: A Good Beginning

One of the most masterful pieces of work in the universe is the human body. It is definitely the most masterful and the most complex thing ever directly encountered by man. Man has sought to understand it from the beginning, but with limited success. That process is still going on and with all the skills of modern science there is still much to learn. The massive research organizations, hospitals, and millions of individual medical efforts combined spend billions annually and still what we know is dwarfed by what we don't know.

I suppose there are some that would take exception to this statement because after completing medical school, internship, and a great deal of pharmacological orientation they feel they have learned just about all there is to know.

Perhaps they did learn about all that has been taught. But the study environment is only learning what others have learned and are passing on. New learning, through experience, observation and inspiration, leads us forward toward truth and knowledge.

After what I have seen in my lifetime and the experience I have had with my own illnesses, I am convinced that man will never discover a significant amount of the Master Creator's knowledge.

1

Each of us has the responsibility for our own health. We grow up with our own bodies and we need to accept them and care for them in order to have good health. To do this we must know our bodies and be fully aware of our individual differences, our strengths, weaknesses, and susceptibilities.

Many people are so unfortunate as to take little or no interest in health and healing until adulthood and the onset of serious illness. I implore the reader to give the next generation (probably your children) a break. Help care for them and teach them what you know about healthy living. It will most assuredly enhance their health and happiness.

This part of the book is devoted to looking at the developmental stages in a person's life and how these stages impact health.

At each stage of development there are many things one needs to learn about. Ultimately, this will enable a person to intelligently select treatment that will be simple and effective.

The world we live in is so strongly oriented to making money that natural health and healing is given too little attention. We are also lazy about our own care and tend to be disconnected from good health care until confronted with some form of serious illness or dysfunction.

This book spends considerable time and effort defining and explaining the many obstacles and problems that will be confronted in seeking individual health care, Understanding the problems and avoiding the obstacles will simplify your efforts to establish a good health care program.

The young and uninformed will be in special need of your help.

Morris "J" Llewellyn

CHAPTER 1: Before Birth

Before birth we are at the mercy of parental care and chance. Birth marks a new beginning. Whether one is agnostic, Christian, Jewish, or affiliated with one of the many eastern religions is of importance so far as prenatal influence is concerned. However, with this in mind, we are all aware of how parents influence the bodies of their children during the fetal period and early in life.

Genetics are a given, but the behavior of a parent does bear heavy influence on the health of the newborn. Recent experience with drug addicts, alcohol, tobacco, and diet bear this out.

We are learning new things all the time and we must bear the responsibility of learning to care for our selves and our children in order to be healthy and get maximum service from our bodies. It is up to parents to give children the best start possible. Regardless of our nursing, attendant medical help, or early influences at birth, we are in a sense on our own. Our genetic gifts are in place and, per current technology, pretty much unalterable.

The potential power and capacity of one's immune system is established at birth. How long we make that immune system last or how fast we destroy it can be varied a great deal by our own behavior. For so long as we live,

5

we will be with this body. How we care for it will determine how long it lasts.

CHAPTER 2: CHILDHOOD

Childhood is a time when one is totally at the mercy of parents. Childhood can be (should be) a time of learning, fun, spiritual growth and good physical development.

A child starts life with a new body, new mind, new brain, and a confident innocence that deserves guidance into a world of beauty and promise. This gift is the simple solution to a healthy start in life and the parents are the only ones that can provide it.

In concept, I know this is an absolute truth. In reality, I know this is the goal of most noble and righteous parents. I also know that there are many obstacles to achieving this goal. Some of the obstacles are natural in nature and are a part of life. Various types of handicaps, some disease, and hardships imposed upon some parents and children alike make things difficult.

I have noticed that in the natural difficulties that come in life there are some compensating factors that work wonders for people with problems. Sometimes there is a resilience, especially in children, that comes with disabilities. It seems as though God is watching and will help. Parents that seek to solve their own problems seem to find help and seem to have good results in family life.

7

There are some social agencies that offer worthwhile help. If you need them, use them for the good of the children.

I have been accused of being an optimist, and a softie. However, when there is neglect, abuse, and ignorance involved, I have often been called a hard ass pessimist. I have no patience with unnecessary nonsense like abuse, ignorance and evil. I think we should encourage all social agencies and police groups to adopt the same attitudes I have and my reasons are for promoting long-term health for our children.

I reiterate, however, there is no substitute for a real parent who is willing and able to provide proper guidance and upbringing.

Am I getting carried away a bit? I don't think so because the parent is the only one that can do the right job for the child. I.e., usher the child into the world prepared and headed in the right direction. What are the Simple Solutions for young children's health? And, what will assure their good health, short and long term?

1. Breast feed, if possible, up to one year. This practice establishes better natural immunity in the child. Some psychiatrists believe this practice offers other benefits such as self confidence and a feeling of closeness to the mother.

2. Provide a clean and healthful environment, as smoke free and pollen free as possible. Second hand cigarette smoke is dangerous and burdensome to all people. It is especially so for children.

3. Love and comforting (or the lack of it) strongly influences the physical and psychological health of children. Babies need to be cuddled and caressed. These influences can affect the health of a person throughout life.

4. Establish a good relationship with a pediatrician or a family doctor ahead of time. I.e., don't wait for an illness before selecting a doctor.

Be the good parent by knowing the above and assist them in the following when needed:

Know a good Pediatrician who understands and uses both Medical and Naturopathic healing methods. Coordinate with this doctor the child's health needs. The parent can usually detect symptoms indicating needs in: Allergies, Skin disorders, Hearing, Vision, Nutrition and Supplements. The child will need help from the parent to do this. As the child grows he will become aware of his own needs and communicate them to a receptive parent.

Morris "J" Llewellyn

CHAPTER 3: EARLY ADULTHOOD

At the beginning of this chapter I want to remind the reader that, as the title implies, the purpose of the book is to identify simple solutions for good health. There are two terrific impediments to achieving this purpose. We must overcome them to achieve a healthy life.

First is the proliferation of false and bad information to those who are not yet well informed. People of any age can be poorly informed for a number of reasons but for the purposes of this chapter I will focus on the younger group. The greatest danger for a young person is to not have an effective mentor. Many people are thrust into society at an early age, often when they begin school, with no knowledge of social sense or rules. This especially applies to common sense about health. An effective mentor, hopefully parents, will teach the young person (age 5 to adult) to come to them with questions about anything new or anything not fully understood.

To be an effective mentor is one of the most difficult tasks in human relations. The importance and the value of this task is greatly under estimated. Our children's social education must be supplemented at every level. Schools don't do this and in my opinion they cannot. Proper guidance in a young person's life will help them adopt healthy habits, teach them to be law abiding and compassionate citizens, and it will show them the road to a healthy and successful life.

I have had many people express their inability to be a successful mentor. We have all most likely seen examples of poor results. The one that haunts me most is the parent and the child appearing on a national TV show screaming into each others face about who is in charge and what their family roles should be. If, from the beginning, the child understands truth and consequences and is held responsible for his own behavior such problems will not develop. How is this accomplished? The mentor can NEVER put any subject off limits for discussion and investigation. The mentor can point out consequences but should never lay a guilt trip on the youngster. Always be upbeat and positive especially about future possibilities.

The second major impediment to achieving our purpose of finding simple solutions for good health is apathy and ignorance. As the cliche indicates, you can lead a thirsty horse to water but he may choose not to drink.

There are too many people who do not seek knowledge and understanding about their own health until they are confronted by a serious health breakdown. This is a big mistake that can cause pain, grief, and possible death. All people should know about the many alternatives available for different kinds of health care. And they should understand their own individual susceptibilities.

When one advances from early adulthood properly educated and trained to use good health practices, that young person will be healthier and happier throughout life. Such a person will understand the values of prevention through avoiding exposure to disease, practicing clean health habits, following a proper diet, and observation of safety rules. Statistics bear out that the young are vulnerable to such things as AIDS, STD, suicide, and accidents.

Proper training at an early stage of life may be the single most important factor in health. However, eventually, we will all suffer some health problems. Some of the following chapters which will get into curing short term illness, healing long term illness and achieving good health and long life. Remember, the best known treatment for any disease or ailment is avoidance. Since the primary purpose of this book is to find simple solutions, I must point out that avoidance is the simplest and most effective.

Morris "J" Llewellyn

PART II: MEETING THE CHALLENGE

This entire book is written from an adult perspective. However, Part 1 is oriented to preparing the young and uninformed for information coming in the following chapters which is progressively more complex and deals with situations that sometimes interfere with approaches to natural healing.

Impediments imposed on health and healing are imposed by the system itself.

The following chapters in Part II will examine Medicine versus Natural Healing, Cures versus Healing, God's role in establishing man's rules for good health. Man's own internal healing capability and simple God-given things that promote health. These things are under fire from various places and we will see that they need to be preserved.

Everyone needs to examine and understand these things before they can take charge of personal health care. Such an understanding will make self treatment plans effective in many situations.

Establishing simple health plans for one's self will be discussed in Part III.

A good place to start in this part of the book is the physical/meta physical. We have had scriptures before we had organized medical science. We open with chapter 4, what God has said about the health of man.

Morris "J" Llewellyn

CHAPTER 4: GOD ON HEALTH

Students of scripture all know that man has suffered much physical torment since the fall of Adam. Examples through the ages are leprosy, the plagues of Egypt, repetitions of the black plague, AIDS and many other modern day illnesses. We accept this as part of the condition of mortality and as part of the testing and learning process of life. Why does God give us both disease and healing? God's purpose is complex and beyond our complete understanding as stated in Isaiah 55: 8-9. "8. For my thoughts are not your thoughts, neither are your ways my ways, saith the Lord. 9. For as the heavens are higher than the earth, so are my ways higher than your ways, and my thoughts than your thoughts."

It is, however, obvious that he wants us to be strong, productive, intelligent and worthy of salvation.

God guides and directs us but does not remove us from the learning experience. As we learn and become more effective in obeying the commandments we become more capable of receiving His help, which is given freely. Having good health makes it more likely that we will have the energy to excel in all that God commands. He has provided guidance and help in all our needs, including health. The help comes through prayer, revelation, inspiration, and scriptures. These sources provide us with much

17

wisdom and practical guidance; more than has been produced by the research of man. It is the purpose of this article to summarize some of this God-given guidance on health.

I refer to scriptures that range from the Old Testament, to the New Testament, and to LDS (Mormon scripture). The purpose is to give perspective to the time frames involved. God has always communicated for the purpose of helping mankind. LDS scripture is used because it is organized and covers the most recent time frame.

It does not matter if you are in any way affiliated with a religion that uses these scriptures. Let the information conveyed stand on its own merit. If you use these guidelines to establish your own health care philosophy, you will be in line with current science and your health will benefit immensely.

But first, please heed these words about "commentary" on scripture. There have been books of commentary written about scriptures and church doctrines. Such commentary should not be considered as authoritative or as important as the original scripture and doctrine. Only appropriate ecclesiastical authority can give absolute definition to scripture. With that in mind, commentary can be effectively used as a guideline for expanded study and thought. The commentary in this article is intended to do only that. And remember, each person is entitled to his own inspiration.

Since the beginning, God's relationship with mortal man has involved disease, sickness, afflictions and famine as well as health, healings and deliverance from all kinds of problems.

Sample references of health related scriptures:

Leviticus 11, The Lord reveals the living things that may or may not be used for food. This guidance is related to what is considered clean or unclean. He commands Israel to be holy and clean.

Leviticus 12 dwells on purification, child birth, and circumcision.

Lev. 13 and 14 revealed, to the people, how to identify and control leprosy.

Lev. 15 gives much detailed information to people of that time on avoiding contamination by disease.

In Exodus 15: 23-27 The Lord provides fresh water and healing.

In Deuteronomy 7: 15 The Lord takes away all sickness. Deut. 23 provides instruction on sanitation.

Deut. 28 shows involvement of The Lord in use of disease, plagues, and every aspect of physical and mental health for punishment and reward; a good example of His involvement from the beginning of religious history.

NOTE OF EXPLANATION: "D&C = Sections of the Doctrine & Covenants of the LDS (Mormon) faith. Other references not from the Old or New Testaments come from the Book of Mormon."

Alma 9:22 demonstrates the hand of The Lord in "famine, sickness and all manner of diseases." Alma 15: 3-11 demonstrates the power of the mind to cause illness and, conversely, to heal. It also demonstrates the involvement of The Lord in healing through faith and prayer (a method recently given credence by some medical doctors). D&C 89: 18-21 gives the promise of great health and knowledge to those who obey the commandments of God. The foregoing references are made to give perspective to God's involvement over time, and, to show a small portion of what God does for us health wise. These are only a few of many scriptures which refer to God's constant involvement in the welfare of mankind. We have been given much advise and guidance, but do we use it?

After almost 7000 years man has not yet learned how to avoid conflict and dilemma. 2 Timothy, chapter 3 foretells one of the better accounts of the perilous times of the last days. Verse seven "Ever learning, and never able to come to the knowledge of the truth" depicts man's effort in many fields including health. Much of the disease and pestilence of earlier times has been overcome only to be replaced by plagues of our own time. We struggle with AIDS, Alzheimer's disease, Cancer, Arthritis, Heart Disease, Diabetes and many elusive viruses.

We are lost in some of these efforts to heal. Why? Perhaps it is because man is too caught up in solving the mysteries of the human body and forcing the healing process with drugs while disregarding the commandments and guidance given by God.

Many research groups continue the effort to map the 46 chromosomes, human DNA and the millions of genetic combinations in an attempt to identify markers associated with disease. Isn't it great that all this research has finally discovered how God constructed the cell? Seriously, knowledge is wonderful. It serves humanity well and God promotes the expansion of knowledge by mankind. But even with advanced data processing methods, it could be many years before the completed mapping can be put to meaningful use. After that, how do we determine the treatment methods required by individual differences in constantly changing body chemistries? It seems unreasonable that establishing and maintaining good health need be that complicated. God blessed us with self healing bodies that have great and variable capacities. His laws for human health are simple and have been available to us from the beginning.

Perhaps God's commandments seem too simple. It is the contention of this article, that as simple as they are, the value of God's commandments are self proving. The most recent scripture in our standard works which relates exclusively to health, D&C 89, bears this out. Because it is so short and so meaningful and full of wisdom (it is known as The Word of Wisdom) it is quoted in its entirety. Use it and you will be greatly rewarded.

"Section 89: Revelation given through Joseph Smith the Prophet, at Kirkland, Ohio, February 27, 1833. HC 1: 327-329. As a consequence of the early brethren using tobacco in their meeting, the Prophet was led to ponder upon the matter; consequently he inquired of the Lord concerning it. This revelation, known as the Word of Wisdom, was the result. The first three verses were originally written as an inspired introduction and description of the revelation given to the Prophet.

1. A Word of Wisdom, for the benefit of the council of high priests, assembled in Kirtland, and the church, and also the saints in Zion—

2. To be sent greeting; not by commandment or constraint, but by revelation and the word of wisdom, showing forth the order and will of God in the temporal salvation of all saints in the last days—

3. Given for a principle with promise, adapted to the capacity of the weak and the weakest of all saints, who are or can be called saints."

Verses 1-3 emphasize the simplicity of section 89. It should be understandable by all and is intended as a guide to temporal salvation for all of us in these perilous times. The basic principles are given here with the promise of salvation. However, many of us tend to interpret health rules in such a way as to accommodate our current behavior. We should do the opposite by embracing these principles and seeking all of the intended meaning, looking for all healthful behavior that might come within the principle given. God has admonished us to do just that, to think for ourselves, to not require finite instruction in everything we do. It would be good to review section 58:26 which states "for behold it is not meet (appropriate) that I should command in all things; for he that is compelled in all things, the same is a slothful and not a wise servant; wherefore he receives no reward." Also, Matthew 24:45-51 warns to be a faithful and wise servant; do not procrastinate to do good lest you reap the evil consequence.

"4.   Behold, verily, thus saith the Lord unto you: In consequence of evils and designs which do and will exist in the hearts of conspiring men in the last days, I have warned you, and forewarn you, by giving unto you this word of wisdom by revelation—

5. That inasmuch as any man drinketh wine or strong drink among you, behold, this is not good, neither meet in the sight of your Father, only in assembling your selves together to offer up your sacraments before him.

6. And behold, this should be wine, yea, pure wine of the grape of the vine, of your own make.

7. And, again, strong drinks are not for the belly, but for the washing of your bodies.

8. And again, tobacco is not for the body, neither for the belly, and is not good for man, but is an herb for bruises and all sick cattle, to be used with judgment and skill.

9. And again, hot drinks are not for the body or belly."

Verses 4-9 are plain enough for most to understand. However, it is interesting to note how the warning of the evils and the designs of conspiring men in the last days coincide with the powerful marketing of alcohol, tobacco and drugs (legal and illegal). Much of the given advice in these verses had no scientific basis when first given. But it is now such common knowledge that the large body of scientific data now available need not be quoted to prove the harmful effects of many commonly used products. Tobacco, alcohol, and many drugs not only do immediate harm to the user but can also cause great harm to unborn children of the users. All addicting products should not be used. Coffee, many teas, and many soda pop drinks have been identified as harmful, especially if used in large quantities. If a product is addicting, users usually consume large amounts. We need to be vigilant to identify and avoid such products. It is not just the product in hot drinks that is harmful. If too hot when taken, the heat will destroy needed natural bacteria in the mouth and the digestive system, not to mention possible burns.

A warning against the use of strong drink is given anciently in the Old Testament. Proverbs 20-1: "Wine is a mocker, and strong drink is raging:

and whosoever is deceived thereby is not wise." And an excellent account of the evils of drunkenness is given in proverbs 23: 29-35.

The guidance given in The Word of Wisdom is well supported by earlier scriptures. Only a few of many are noted here. Some are repetitive but are noted for the benefit of those who need proof of God's continued effort to warn and help us, and for those who might want more validation of Joseph Smith's revelations.

"10. And again, verily I say unto you, all wholesome herbs God hath ordained for the constitution, nature, and use of man—

11. Every herb in the season thereof, and every fruit in the season thereof; all these to be used with prudence and thanksgiving.

12. Yea, flesh also of beasts and of the fowls of the air, I, the Lord, have ordained for the use of man with thanksgiving; nevertheless they are to be used sparingly;

13. And it is pleasing unto me that they should not be used, only in times of winter, or of cold, or famine.

14. All grain is ordained for the use of man and of beasts, to be the staff of life, not only for man but for the beasts of the field, and the fowls of heaven, and all wild animals that run or creep on the earth;

15. And these hath God made for the use of man only in times of famine and excess of hunger.

16. All grain is good for the food of man; as also the fruit of the vine; that which yieldeth fruit, whether in the ground or above the ground—

17. Nevertheless, wheat for man, and corn for the ox, and oats for the horse, and rye for the fowls and for swine, and for all beasts of the field, and barley for all useful animals, and for mild drinks, as also other grain."

Does God promote vegetarianism? Promote, probably yes. Command, No. The concept of using a plant oriented diet versus using meat has been a part of scripture since the beginning. Even in the first chapter of Genesis 1: 29-30, at the time of organizing the creation, God commanded the use of seeds, the fruit of trees, and green herbs. And again in Genesis 9: 3-4, Noah and his sons were reminded that all living things are for the benefit of man with comment which promotes the green herb and forbids the eating of blood.

Compared to the diet of the average American, the diet suggested here is much more natural and favors vegetarianism. Verses 10-15 are very direct and clear. In recent years even the American Cancer Society, The Institute of National Health, and many doctors have begun to recommend low fat diets and natural foods as a means of avoiding illness. A good portion of naturopathic medicine is based on the use of herbs and a diet of fruit and vegetables. Health oriented diets suggest vegetable sources for most of our essential oils and proteins such as beans, olive oil and flax seed oil. Verse 12 gives permission to use the flesh of animals and fowl. Then verse 13 indicates that the Lord would be pleased if we do not use meat except in times of special need. Verses 14 and 15 make it clear that we should not use wild animals except in emergency situations. Verses 16 and 17 are explicit about using fruits, vegetables and grains. Grains have been used as the staff of life from the beginning. It is interesting how these products are used extensively by health professionals in scientifically balanced diets. To name a few products that are now recommended in the best natural diets: Whole grain breads and cereals, various sprouts, green juices from wheat grass and barley grass and health drinks made from grain. Cruciferous vegetables, carrots, beets, and potatoes are considered special health foods.

"18.   And all saints who remember to keep and do these sayings, walking in obedience to the commandments, shall receive health in their navel and marrow to their bones;

19.   And shall find wisdom and great treasures of knowledge, even hidden treasures;

20.   And shall run and not be weary and shall walk and not faint.

21.   And I, the Lord, give unto them a promise, that the destroying angel shall pass by them, as the children of Israel, and not slay them. Amen."

Verses 18-21 are less specific than prior verses but, if taken literally, may carry even greater significance. Perhaps we need to look for the detail here. The message given here, as applies to health, is partially implied. But the obvious message is that if we observe the specific instructions given and obey all of God's commandments we will experience dimensions of wisdom and health beyond our greatest expectations. Just a few examples of how God's other commandments impact health: Some of the greatest destroyers of mental and physical health are stress, envy, hate, covetousness, anger, guilt, fatigue, selfishness and gluttony, to name a few. If only the ten commandments were observed there would be a great impact on these destroyers of health.

Just a few additional LDS scriptures which describe the effects of behavior on health: D&C Section 59 discusses the benefits of the fast, sacrifice, and obedience to the commandments. D&C Section 82 further points out the benefits of obedience to the commandments; the Lord saying "I am bound when ye do what I say". He also instructs us to do good and seek to help our neighbors. D&C Section 88 explores justice, law, intelligence, light and truth. D&C 88: 124 "Cease to be idle; cease to be unclean; cease to find fault one with another; cease to sleep longer than is needful; retire to thy bed early, that ye may not be weary; arise early, that your bodies and your minds may be invigorated."

God assures us that we can have health and happiness. With such guidance, we have the power to choose a healthy life. It is folly to destroy good health with bad habits then seek a doctor to restore it. Prevention is the best cure and we have now been shown the way. However, if health need be restored, it is often possible by adopting good habits, obeying the commandments, taking control of one's life and using the help of a good doctor. But remember, healing requires the participation of the patient.

CHAPTER 5: POWER HEALING

Nothing God had to say about health conflicts with good principles of healing. This chapter is about what a person can do on his own. It is part of my personal story about healing.

In April of 1991 exploratory surgery revealed that I had inoperable cancers in the liver and the mesentery of the stomach. An oncologist ordered me to his office to begin chemotherapy immediately with the promise of 20% chance of success. Success meant a probable survival of two years. I opted out. He told me I had six months to live and noted at the bottom of my hospital release papers "This patient refuses treatment in the face of certain death."

A few months ago, I had a complete body CAT scan. There was no sign of cancer. This chapter will relate how I learned about power healing.

Power Healing is an extension of the natural healing process. This is a simple definition. However, it's application is not so simple because most people, and many doctors, do not understand the true nature of healing.

Healing must be differentiated from curing. Healing is a natural process that takes place in the body. Curing is a process that is usually imposed by a foreign substance. It may promote healing by killing bacteria. To demonstrate the difference, my best example is the poor pig. A dead pig cannot be healed, but his flesh can be cured. I.e. cured ham or bacon.

One must understand the healing process before applying the principles of Power Healing.

What qualifies me to make strong assertions on this subject? It's the experience I have had in healing my own ailments and the extensive study of healing methods. This article is the story of how I have stayed alive by learning the true nature of healing.

Many of the people who become ill want a quick fix yet know nothing about healing. Medical doctors are usually pressed to produce results and they do their best to serve their patients demands. Sometimes it works and sometimes it doesn't. Most of the doctors, to which I refer, have medical knowledge that far exceeds my own. I hold no medical license and do not provide medical advice or treatment to anyone. The self experimentation and treatments I have indulged in have been based on much study of research already done. None of these ventures have ever involved anything harmful nor have they encroached upon "medical domain."

Much of poor health and healing has to do with life style. With the exception of serious fetal damage, I believe life style even surpasses genetics as the primary control element in human health.

In my very early years I was strong and healthy. This was most likely due to my life on the farm involving long hours of work, good simple food, clean water, fresh air, and a happy simplistic life. During my stint in the Navy, a few years in college, ten years in the Foreign Service, and another ten years in a stressful corporate environment my life style changed a great deal. At the age of 40 I had acquired a case of moderate hypertension. Being an athletic type with lots of energy I was not alarmed when my company doctor sent me for a complete medical exam. The cardiologist at the clinic insisted I start medication. I did so. I was started on a typical treatment beginning with diuretics. This helped temporarily but as is often the case beta blockers were added then when high blood pressure continued other drugs were added. After a while I was on five different kinds of drugs for a simple case of hypertension.

Back then I was ignorant about proper health care and, like most people in our culture, totally reliant upon a medical system well trained in drug use and untrained in health care or natural healing. Had I known, I could have resolved my own problem with life style modifications such as eliminating tobacco use, cutting or eliminating use of alcohol, eating proper food like I had on the farm, reducing work hours to 50 per week, and taking a restful vacation with my family. I did none of these. I only followed the cardiologists instructions and had a heart attack at age 42.

The company ambulance rushed me to the local community hospital where I was put in intensive care. My regular doctor was called but he refused to come because he was with another patient who was dying as the result of heart attack and kidney failure.

Little did I know it, but that was my lucky day! The only other doctor available, and willing to take my case, was an older fellow considered by many to be a cranky old coot. He was really a genius with specialties in cardiology, atomic medicines, and sports medicine. Lucky for me sports medicine was his passion. He had almost died with a heart attack of his own caused by extreme obesity. He had obviously survived his cardiac problem and had adopted many of the dietary and exercise ideas he had been pushing with the athletes. Because of his fantastic progress he had become thin and energetic, almost fanatic about diet, eating little meat and no sugar. He had converted to the new life style so completely that he had written and published two books on sports medicine incorporating his own ideas on life style. At the time he was considered very radical by his peers but today he looks real smart. It was my good fortune to get him as a doctor.

On our first visit he threw down my cover and looked at my pot belly saying "that damn thing has to go!" Well it went and I survived. However, there had been sufficient damage. I used nitroglycerin for almost a year to ward off extreme arrhythmia. The attack left me with permanent mitral valve prolapse. That doctor saved my life by getting me off drugs that are commonly used for cardiac patients. He knew that the body works as a unit, that there is a need to achieve balance and unity in the body. He knew that the body has terrific self healing potential and that it is the responsibility of the patient to encourage those self healing functions of the body by giving it the things it needs. What we did back then was only a glimmer of what I now call Power Healing.

Shortly after this experience I left that part of the country and gradually lost track of that great doctor. Little did I know it then but my experience with health problems and Power Healing had only begun.

About that time I received word that my mother had cancer. Prior to that time I had no special interest in deadly diseases and knew nothing about genetic disorders or immunity. I later found out that every death in my mother's family, for two generations, had been caused by cancer.

Unfortunately my life style drifted a bit off its new course but I still felt good. I even thought my health was safe. I never went back to using tobacco or alcohol but I gradually gained weight which was the result of relaxed dietary rules and less exercise. At an earlier age I was a boxer. I sparred three times a week. On the other three days of my routine I skipped rope, ran, and lifted weights. My fighting weight was 147 pounds. Over the years I learned that I functioned well between 160 and 170 pounds, with exercise, beyond that weight I knew I had a problem. I mention this detail because it is a significant part of Power Healing to know yourself.

We have been endowed with complex internal communication systems. If you listen and become aware of self, your body tells you much of what you need to know about your own health. The signals are breathing patterns, ability to relax, digestion, and various kinds of pain. If only we would listen and react accordingly we could avoid lots of difficulty.

I am more aware of my body needs now than I was then. The spirit of reckless optimism is one of the curses of youth, always ignoring threatening signs of danger.

I managed well for fifteen years. Then, at age 57, I started to feel bad and gradually became so dysfunctional that I had to retire at age 58. My plans to conquer the world came crashing down as I searched for a diagnosis and cure. I went from one highly recommended clinic to another seeking answers. I was finally given several tentative answers including the embarrassing recommendation for psychotherapy. I was desperate enough to try anything. There proved to be no need in this area. A note of caution to anyone who has a difficult illness to diagnose: psychogenic illness is a remote possibility worthy of exploration but it is more likely to be used as a way out by a stumped or incompetent doctor.

Depending on which specialist was consulted, I was at the beginning stages of Myasthenia Gravis, Multiple Sclerosis, Food Allergies, Arthritis, and a variety of Arthritic disorders such as Lupus and Sjogren's Syndrome. It was a sorry situation. I was disabled and couldn't get a confirmed diagnosis.

At this point I came to a startling realization. I was alone—strictly on my own so far as health care was concerned. Rather than giving up, as many people do, I went more and more into studies of the body and into self administered health care. I was compelled to continue working with several doctors because I needed their certification for disability retirement. This led to continued, almost endless, testing. After more than two years it became evident, and finally officially concluded, that my illness was a combination of Rheumatoid Arthritis and Sjogren's Syndrome with Central Nervous System involvement. The prognosis for this disease is dire, continued progression, the drying up of tear ducts and salivary glands, eventual blindness, development of Lymphoma and death.

The conventionally educated medical doctors have no knowledge of what causes these diseases. They offer no cures. However, they give intensive treatments to millions of people in similar circumstances. The treatments are oriented toward reduction of inflammation and pain. Short term treatments are usually helpful but long term results can be disastrous.

At last I had the diagnosis which helped me to direct my self healing efforts. The problems with glands and eyes had been abated if not avoided. However, at age 64, I did discover a large lump in my stomach one morning while working out. I consented to exploratory surgery. I almost expected the results. I had a large cleaved small cell lymphoma at the intermediate stage. I also had six small tumors in my liver. My surgeon was a good one. He had enough common sense to not mutilate me in an effort to remove all tumors. They were too advanced and critically located for removal. He put me back together and recommended the services of an oncologist.

I was concerned but for some reason I was not fearful nor did I panic. I realized that I had peaked out. My disease had reached its pinnacle and I now had to have my final battle with it. Could I win? I didn't know. My relatives and friends all advised me to follow the advise of the oncologist. He made it easy for me to refuse his services. He seemed anxious to instill fear, panic and urgency. He literally ordered me to be in his office for chemotherapy staging as soon as I was released from the hospital. His prognosis for the treatment was 20% probability for my recovery. He left me with the opinion that he merely wanted a fee before I died. I still have a copy of his final hospital report. His final handwritten subscript was "This patient refuses my treatment in the face of certain death!" He later called me at home urging me to take chemotherapy treatments. I refused and asked him how much time he thought I had. "Six months" was his reply. That was in April of 1991, ten years ago. I had full body CAT scans several months ago which revealed no cancer activity.

I expect this story to end at around age 90 when I will die from some unexpected cause other than Sjogren's syndrome or cancer.

What does the end of my life's story have to do with Power Healing? Everything! That is the story of Power Healing.

SUGGESTIONS

What is needed for successful Power Healing:

First, one must have an attitude. Don't be a blind follower. Be confident and know as much as possible about what you are doing. Learn and be self reliant but get all the help you can.

The tools of healing are God given. Healing only takes place in the body. A good doctor understands that the secrets to healing are within the patient. He can help the healing process by manipulation, stimulation, and repairs but he cannot heal, the patient must do that.

There are many levels of intelligence in the body other than conscious brain function. If you doubt this ponder the workings and nature of cells, the process of miosis and mitosis then the continuing process of cell differentiation and redifferentiation. In other words how does a cell decide whether it will be a part of the toe nail or the eye or the heart or something else? How do body parts know when to stop growing?

Also consider the many organic functions that are continuous and regulated to vary according to need. As examples consider digestion, breathing, heart beat and circulation, lymphatic flow, the variety of nervous systems and senses and the variations in brain chemistry and function.

The importance of this in healing is that all of the above can be influenced and sometimes controlled by you, the patient. And how can this be done? By applications of Feedback, Meditation, Visualization, Prayer, and various sensory perceptions. With practice a person can get very good at it. And with practice a person can develop dimensions of Power Healing that satisfy special requirements.

To realize success in healing all the energies involved must be cared for. That is where diet plays a role. And in addition to diet there is scientific supplementation, proper diagnostics, energy transfer, and energy balance. The science of kinesiology can be used to accomplish much of this. The crude form of this is muscle testing. In our high tech age some naturopathic doctors have computerized electronic devises that can do this very effectively. The electronic devises are good because they eliminate the subjectivity that gets involved in manual testing.

The entire book on this subject is not yet complete but these guidelines should be enough direction for anyone wishing to pursue the benefits of Power Healing. If you need additional help where do you go?

Many naturopathic doctors and osteopathic doctors get involved in at least some of these techniques. They exist in most states. Only about ten states are open to the many health treatment modalities available today. The health industry is just beginning to wake up to the fact that the standard American medical approach to healing is limited and it is not the only good health care available. The Holistic Health Directory published by New Age Magazine lists 150 different health treatment modalities. This includes a listing of 6000 practitioners in the United States.

The state of Washington is the best place to look for a good pool of doctors that use alternative treatments.

To find a medical practitioner contact:

American Holistic Medical Association
2002 Eastlake Avenue East
Seattle, WA 98102 tel. (206) 322-6842

American Association of Naturopathic Physicians
P.O. Box 20386
Seattle, WA 98102 tel. (206) 323-7610

CHAPTER 6: THE DILEMMA OF LONG TERM ILLNESS

Chapter 6 points to some of the many problems we face in the medical world itself.

We really need to understand what's wrong, what to avoid, what to use and what we can develop on our own.

THE DILEMMA OF LONG TERM ILLNESS shows us some of the weaknesses in the medical system, who is involved and who is affected. We will see how good medicine is victimized. As potential patients, we must know how to protect ourselves.

The average person's thoughts are likely consumed by fear and panic when confronted with a diagnosis of terminal illness, especially if it is cancer. Yet beyond the fears of those intimately associated with these diseases, there exists one of the largest dilemmas of our time.

We have no cure for cancer and too few useful treatments for many long-term diseases. As a society we are in a bind. Uninformed patients are using physicians who are indoctrinated with dogma that is wrong. All this is perpetuated by misdirected research and greedy profiteers in the pharmaceutical and health care industries. This situation is deeply imbedded in current culture. What are physicians and victimized patients to do? We can't tolerate the current situation so how do we fix it? Who will be powerful and honest enough to buck the system? I call this situation a real dilemma and as a society we need to deal with the following related issues..

Victims and their families carry the heaviest burdens of frustration, pain, and death but this dilemma bears heavily on us all. We all need to be socially and politically involved to help solve this problem. We should make use of our government representatives to represent our wishes. Read on to see how some groups are involved and why their involvement feeds and perpetuates this harmful dilemma. Then, very possibly, our involvement will help to bring about a resolution.

THE ROLE OF DOCTORS AND MEDICAL INSTITUTIONS

Doctors and medical institutions have perpetuated the greatest part of this dilemma having been caught up in a situation created almost 100 years ago by unscrupulous profiteers. And now HMO's contribute their bit of confusion by adding new dimensions of administrative control that contribute little to successful research and actually pose a threat to the welfare of patients. Their basic purpose is to impose cost constraints intended to assure greater profits for the HMO. This is infuriating, dangerous, anti American, and an obstacle to the progress we need. HMO'S are only the latest obstacle to be placed between the doctor and the patient.

I have personally experienced a near breakdown in the patient doctor relationship. Sixty five years ago I was a very small boy. I was very ill with a series of viral diseases and could have easily died, but I didn't. I lived in the country about six miles from the nearest town where my doctor lived. He used to come to my house on a horse or in an old model T Ford. His medical education and techniques were not the best even for his time. The best back then wasn't very good. None of us were very prosperous then for a number of reasons. Probably the most compelling reason being the great Depression. Money was hard to come by. The number one purpose of several people who were involved in my case was to get me well. After many months I did recover.

The medical doctor, the old lady herbalist, the Indian spiritual healer, my religious leader and my parents all put forth their best efforts to bring about my healing. That was the last healing effort I remember in which payment was not a primary issue and which was not monitored or controlled by some organization. Since that time I have seen the personal relationship between doctor and patient dwindle. In some areas HMO's have delivered the final death blow to this essential relationship in a true healing process.

The current dilemma bears heavily on medical doctors. Some of them function fully aware that most treatments for cancer and other ailments are inadequate while others just follow guidelines established by organizations. The AMA and other regulatory medical organizations, such as state medical boards, control physicians with an iron fist. We the public should not put up with it. Doctors are already beyond being able to do much about it. They need our help and we need better treatments that make sense. Commonly prescribed Chemotherapy and Radiation treatments are either harmful or ineffective. Organized medicine and research need to know and recognize that standardized medicine in this country only represents one of many treatment modalities for disease. The powerful AMA and state medical boards have hamstrung doctors and the public by using their powerful lobbies to establish laws making the practice of other methods of treating disease unlawful in some areas. If you think the evil dictators in the world are bad, compare them to the people who control our medicine and drugs. This is an invasion of our freedom and we should not put up with it.

Establishment medicine is out of line. However, we should remember that most medical doctors are victimized in this situation. Many people blame medical doctors unjustly for horrible treatments and poor results. Cancer treatments are a good example. But in many ways medical doctors are dictated to from the day they leave high school. The medical training they receive is geared to the profitability of privately owned research organizations and pharmaceutical companies. If the medical schools are not owned by the controlling interests, they gain a contracted control by providing the drugs and tools required for successfully conducting a medical school. Graduating students often believe they now know all there is to know about treating illness. This is one of the biggest lies in the universe! A part of the Hippocratic oath taken by doctors is to first do no harm when they are issued a license to "practice" medicine, a heavy responsibility for anyone with a conscience. And good doctors will "practice" with good judgment and within the areas of their knowledge and experience. This should include other information that may become available to them about the unique condition of a particular patient. Since patients are all unique the doctor needs to know his patient. Building confidence and trust between patient and doctor is a great step toward healing. Perhaps medical doctors suffer the greatest challenge of all when they realizes they have been limited by their own education and that they may be puppets of their own medical association.

THE ROLE OF RESEARCH

Research is the key to new knowledge. God knows we need it! There are appearances of some success in very technical areas such as genetic research, hormonal and dietary research along with many areas of promise shown in alternative health care. One of our big problems is that racketeering and profiteering still abound in medical research and consequently no cancer cure or any other type of cure will ever succeed or even be allowed unless there are handsome profits for those who are in control. There is much collusion between the AMA, FDA, various research organizations, and officials who make the laws and regulations. Perhaps this is just one of the disadvantages of democracy and capitalism. Compared to other systems, it may be worth the trip, but surely, it could be improved upon.

In any event, we need to do much more! We need to make the laws, enforce them and demand much better self-policing by all medical and research organizations. The power of money dominates and has done so in the fields of medical research and education since the establishment of the first medical schools in the United States over 100 years ago..

Large donations allowed the Carnegie and Rockefeller families to dictate to medical schools and everything coming there from. Their dictates, supported by the Flexner Report since 1910, have established the mold for medical schools which still dominates today. These controlling financial interests still exist. They dictate to most of the large research organizations. It is important to remember Rockefeller's well known and published motto, "never give a dollar away unless it comes back with another dollar attached." Has any real altruism ever existed in this situation? Very doubtful!

Now, I have nothing against capitalism, profits, or money. However, when organizations are established, and allowed to perpetuate, for the sole purpose of making billions from a public that is victimized by loss of health and life itself, I believe that the public should arise and demand just treatment.

There is no reason to limit valid research. It should be expanded to include those areas previously denied by the profiteers.

As a reader of this report, I expect you to be doubtful and critical of my statements and implications. I have barely given a glimmer of the entire truth because this brief report cannot relate the many aspects of this situation nor quote the many authentic sources of reliable information. If you are interested, and I hope you are, please refer to the two following sources:

Racketeering In Medicine - The Suppression of Alternatives by James P. Carter, MD, Dr. P.H. Published by Hampton Roads Publishing Company, Inc. Copyright 1992, 1993. This book gives extreme, factual, detailed reports too extensive for quoting here, but worth reading.

Tainted Truth by Cynthia Crossen - Published by Simon & Schuster - copyright 1994

If you are not afraid to find out, and want to do something about it, this is a must read.

Read the above books. If you are interested there are many other sources of good information. I especially like the periodic reports published in news letters by medical doctors who have seen beyond the smoke screen put up by many of their peers and medical organizations such as the AMA, FDA, state medical boards, HMO's and some government regulators. These wonderful doctors that I call "Mavericks" will probably save the profession of health care from the things that are going on in the shadows, things that threaten good doctors and good research. Fortunately there are more of these doctors around than most people realize. Some of my favorite doctors listed below have already published books and papers about various healing methods not routinely taught in medical schools. My favorites are: James Balch, MD, Julian Whitaker, MD, Leo Galland, MD, Dennis Remington, MD, James A. Duke, Phd. Andrew Weil, MD, John A. McDougall, MD, Stephen Sinatra, MD, and David G. Williams, MD.

THE ROLE OF INSURANCE COMPANIES

Insurance companies assume a position which appears to be cooperative and supportive of patients. But they are necessarily motivated by profits and they are involved in the same foul mix of racketeering, profiteering, controlled research, and politics as are other areas of medicine. By necessity insurance operating systems are in bed with medicine, government, and HMO's. It strikes me that if insurance managers are as brilliant and profit oriented as they present themselves to be, stock holders would demand careful consideration of the following facts:

Insurance companies hold the purse strings to a lot of money. This equates to power which could be used to influence many current laws and procedures.

Insurance companies could please many customers and save billions of dollars by NOT forcing people to accept medical treatments when they could choose other treatment modalities.

To prevent double claims, patients should be offered a choice of treatment modalities. Medicine and pharmaceuticals would complain bitterly because this procedure would eliminate some of their easy gravy. However, every time a client chose an alternative to conventional medical treatment many thousands of dollars would be saved for the attendant insurance company. This is not to mention the benefits to the client/patient of much less cost and less pain and suffering. It has been my experience that many illnesses respond better to natural treatments than to modern medicine. This is especially true for long term illnesses such as arthritis, viral diseases, some heart disorders, and many cancers. Compare the costs of chelation therapy to those of heart bypass surgery when each procedure is priced at many thousands of dollars. In addition to the cost consideration, chelation presents no danger and no pain as opposed to great cost, much pain and danger, and a low success rate offered by bypass surgery. There exists a similar comparison in cancer therapies. On a lesser scale the comparison of treatments of viral disease with medicine as opposed to natural treatments, show the natural treatments are more successful at much less cost. Many related studies exist on the Net and in daily news reports.

I have personally found an advantage in using conventional medical techniques for most diagnostics. I then use less invasive, more natural, and more successful modalities for treatment. I have personally had great success with this method in treating arthritis, candida infection, muscle infection, and advanced lymphoma.

Solutions for the many serious health problems actually present opportunities for insurance companies. The insurance industry should "get with it". We could all benefit.

THE ROLE OF PHARMACEUTICAL COMPANIES

The pharmaceutical industry presents many problems to all those involved in any aspect of the this situation. Collectively, this industry presents a great problem to the medical profession, insurance companies, and to informed patients. God help those who are not informed, for they are almost certain to become victims of the system. This problem can be summarized by merely pointing out the fact that pharmaceutical companies aggressively sell anything that will turn a profit. And especially recently, they have become aggressive and skillful in cornering markets and increasing prices to unreasonable levels. The sheer volume of new drugs now available seems to have overwhelmed medical doctors and the FDA seems to have lost its way as protector of the public.

This problem is being recognized by some of the more responsible people who are concerned with health care in the United States. Scott P. Serota, Executive Vice President and Chief Operating Officer at the Blue Cross and Blue Shield Association ran a full page advertisement in the November 8, 1999 issue of NEWSWEEK MAGAZINE highlighting the rising cost of prescription drugs and expressing concern over increased dependence on medications. He points out that much of the demand for, and increased cost of, prescription remedies arises from the drug industries' own marketing programs. There was a time when most of this type of advertising was done only in medical journals. However, in 1998 drug firms spent $1.3 billion promoting products directly to consumers, and it is still going up. That's one reason your drugs cost so much more these days. Another big reason for the growing cost spiral is a rapid influx of new medicines that pass on many additional costs. The FDA accommodated this trend by speeding up its process for approving new drugs.

This has increased demand for pharmaceuticals. It has also created problems for doctors. They have problems keeping up with what drugs are now best for a given treatment. Comprehensive lists of medicines are now made to help doctors choose the most effective drugs for specific conditions. This may entail additional risks for patients.

These lists are included as part of comprehensive plans which encourage doctors to use certain drugs as a part of cost plans. God save us from the involvement of HMO's for their first priority is profit not patient welfare. More than 1000 new drugs are currently in the pipeline to treat cancer and other long term illnesses. Patients beware! There are already many ineffective medical treatments being used today, especially for cancer.

THE ROLE OF GOVERNMENT AND REGULATING ENTITIES

This is where we can become involved. To be effective in this area we have to be tenacious, demanding and persistent. The government is supposed to represent us and protect us (the public). Remember Congress (our representatives) makes the laws. The laws we are considering here are mostly by the FDA. Assuming the FDA has lost its way or sold its soul, we need to press the lawmakers to correct the laws and establish enforcement.

Between the FDA, the AMA, HMO's, insurance companies, pharmaceutical companies, and self regulating medical groups, patients are being misled, abused, and robbed, not only of their money, but their rights and their health..

WHAT ABOUT VICTIMS

Probably the greatest dilemma for most victims is how to deal with the doctor's original diagnosis, "I am sorry but you have cancer." This could be any serious disorder, I use cancer as a good example.

At this point many people lose control. They panic and fall victim to anyone professing the ability to help. If a person having cancer (or other serious disorder) can get past this point, regain self-control, and do some rational thinking, that person may find an appropriate healing method that will save life and restore good health. When evaluating the many treatment options, consider the following:

Except for rare cases there is plenty of time to investigate and decide. Cancer (and other serious disorders) generally develop over time as a result of lifestyle. No significant change will take place overnight or even in a week or so. Victims are often confronted by medical salespersons that want the money up front, but there is no need to panic. In such a case you can probably find better service elsewhere even if the same type of treatment is used. It is not a good sign when more attention is given to the money than is given to the patient.

Remember that pharmaceutical companies exercise way too much influence over organized medicine. They bombard doctors with advertising and new methods for using drugs. This goes way back to the days when the Rockefeller group heavily invested in pharmaceuticals, got control of medical schools, and managed to get in bed with the American Medical Association. Since then, and especially since the use of sulfa drugs and antibiotics during the 1940's, they have managed to convince the United States and much of the world that allopathic medicine (treatment with drugs) was the only legitimate form of health care. This is one of the biggest lies ever perpetrated. Consequently, other health care methods are not widely used though they exist throughout the country and offer some treatments that are far more successful than drug use. I have personally used many of these techniques with great success. Find out about all the alternatives. The better educated you are, the happier and more satisfied you will be. You might even save your own life, as I have saved mine.

If your doctor is put off by your desire to participate in alternative treatment, look for another doctor. A good doctor is not threatened by an educated patient and recognizes that two heads are better than one, especially for something as elusive as cancer. Always remember that prevention is better than cure.

Should anyone try to sell you on the idea that medical practitioners are infallible, please note that according to the statistics of the Institute of Medicine, mistakes made by doctors and other health care workers kill up to 98,000 Americans each year. Don't be hesitant to look around or to be critical.

If you are leaning toward using the standard drug and radiation treatments you should remember that overall cancer treatments for the past 50 years have realized something less than a 50% cure rate. The way I see it, standard medical treatments for cancer equate to a "shot in the dark." That's why I chose to go with natural treatments only. We don't have official statistics on these treatments, but my program worked for me.

It is a lot easier and more cost effective to gain knowledge of natural treatments now before you need to use them. Be sure to read the chapters on establishing your own treatment plan in Part III.

Naturopathic medicine uses many techniques that are natural and do not use prescription drugs. Different naturopathic doctors use many approaches including some of the following, so look around. To name a few methods that are very effective and often not considered in our drug oriented culture: exercise, diet, vitamins used as medicine, massage therapy, homeopathic medicines, energy transfer, and a large variety of mind control techniques. Also Ancient folklore has produced many healing tonics. I have been very successful using cellular manipulation, magnetic power and a variety of detoxification techniques. There are also many other treatments coming from Indian and Oriental cultures. There are doctors in this country who have expert knowledge in administering these treatments.

MY OWN CANCER DILEMMA

I feel justified and compelled to write this article because I have studied natural treatments for ten years. I was driven to study and do self experimentation because every death in my mother's family for two generations was caused by cancer. Eleven years ago I received the jolting news that it was about to be my turn. I agreed to exploratory surgery to get a precise diagnosis. The news was disturbing: a cleaved small cell lymphoma intertwined within the mesentery of my stomach as well as six lesions in my liver. The location of the baseball-sized tumor in my stomach made the cancer inoperable and the six small cancers in my liver was certain evidence that it had metastasized.

At this point I was confronted with my own dilemma. I was not educated in oncology or in standard medical procedures. However, I did have a strong insight into many natural health procedures as a result of personal battles with rheumatoid diseases. I did know about the futility of many treatments for cancer. I discovered that sometimes such treatments are helpful but promote death in the long run. My predicament was not about whether to accept the standard treatment offered but how to discover the natural treatment modality most likely to succeed for me.

My own family was upset to think that I was unwilling to accept, what was in their eyes, the best available medical help.

It is a lonely trip and it takes some courage but you must find out about other available treatments and decide for yourself what is best. I never accepted any chemotherapy or radiation. Over a short period of time I designed my own treatment plan using only natural techniques. It has now been ten years and I am fine.

For help in designing your own treatment plan see Chapter 7 on Finding Your Own Master Healer. And also review Part III for specific products involved. Designing your own treatment plan may sound spooky, especially for the first time and also especially for a deadly disease. I considered a great deal of information and evaluated the advice of many. After a great deal of careful study and review, this complex situation suddenly seemed to have a simple solution. The key to a simple solution is to understand the problem. It is a challenge, it is possible and it can be rewarding.

Morris "J" Llewellyn

CHAPTER 7: FINDING YOUR OWN MASTER

HEALER

The experts have tried to identify how healing takes place from the beginning of time. They have embraced it, studied it, become confounded and cast it aside then started over. They see it and live with it and use it. Yet, today we still struggle to effectively define the process. There is some mystery in most healing. Much healing results from a variety of treatments, while some seems to be spontaneous. I have found the major part of healing to evolve from within the patient. I call this process the MASTER HEALER. I attempt to explain what I have learned about it in this chapter.

The development of various philosophies about healing and the plethora of treatment methods have accumulated over time, prompted by mankind's need and desire to know. We have records of efforts in these areas that go as far back as recognized means of communication. We have developed many treatment methods but our understanding and control of the healing process is still limited.

Discoveries by the ancients have produced some treatments still used today in our country and around the world. And in our time, useful discoveries are being made at an ever increasing rate which help to treat illness and disease. But we still do not understand or control the basic healing process. In our culture we delude ourselves when we use the terms healer and healthcare. Some people call themselves "healer" or "shaman" but, at best, they may influence the process but they do not control it. In our culture, "Healthcare" is a misnomer. Most of what we call healthcare is really disease care. Our medical systems, our medical doctors and our institutions such as hospitals are not trained to know much about health care. We make little or no effort in this direction. Our efforts are directed toward caring for illness and disease as opposed to preventing disease and maintaining good health.

Various systems have developed around the world as a result of efforts to treat disease and understand healing. The never ending search for the true master healing process seems to have been given more attention in cultures other than our own. Western cultures have always given most of the attention to the disease as opposed to the patient. Consequently, the "master healing process" has never been fully defined by us. Various systems have been developed in different cultures by different scientific approaches which has yielded thousands of treatment techniques for various ailments, defined and not defined. Much commonality appears in the results of these efforts even though they were isolated from each other by time, distance and language. Most of these approaches to treatment would be looked upon as non-medical by American medicine, and the purely "AMA" medical group would distance themselves from any approach other than their own. However, the sensibility of good diet, good exercise, good rest, stress management, meaningful lifetime activity, and recognition of individual strengths and weaknesses apply to almost all of these approaches.

These things are the basis of good health regardless of various philosophical approaches to treating illness. It is also noteworthy that nearly all medicines have a common background having been derived from plant sources. They have just been developed in different ways, whether it be the common aspirin or some obscure herbal compound used by jungle natives.

A number of those have been introduced to our own culture in recent years. Even some have found their way into advanced American medicine, such as rauwolfia, an Indian herb used extensively in hypertensive medication, and curare used as powerful anesthesia for some surgery requiring motor paralysis and deep sleep.

I have great respect for doctors of our time who pursue truth in various areas wherever it takes them. They follow a quest for effective health care long after their basic medical training. Some of these doctors now promote blended medicine (taking from other treatments and philosophies and using the best approach to a given health need). They do so because they see effective means of fighting disease. Their number is increasing rapidly as evidenced by many books, clinics and published studies. Two such doctors of renown who have done much to promote all forms of effective treatment are Andrew Weil, M.D. and Deepak Chopra., M.D. I know their work and I listen to them. Their numerous writings reveal much about effective treatments and blended medicine. I recommend that everyone seek this kind of information. It may save your life, not to mention money and endless grief. To give perspective to the current situation it is necessary to note the differences on two levels, the philosophical basis and the many techniques developed from that basis.

Most of the major approaches to treating disease are based on different philosophies. Treatments are so numerous and diverse that it becomes difficult to distinguish between the philosophy and the various specializations within. The American medical approach is a good example having specialties for almost every illness and every age group. The most popular tools are prescription drugs, surgery or psychiatry. These are the mainstays of American medicine. However, some recent movement has been made toward using herbals, vitamins and minerals, exercise and physical therapies. Designed therapies are used broadly for many patients, consequently the primary attention of American medicine is directed toward the disease as opposed to the individual.

Chinese medicine follows a healing system that is as different from mainstream American medicine as the Chinese language is from English. Their methods have endured, according to available records, for 4,500 years. The Materia Medica of She Nong and the Nei Jing established around 200 B.C. set the basic framework for Chinese medicine. Western medicine has become available to the Chinese but they still rely primarily on the Chinese approach. Western physicians target germs. Chinese physicians target forces that are out of balance within the body. Both Western and Chinese rely on medical history and physical exams but that is where commonality ends. The Chinese physician's tools are his senses—what he sees, hears, smells and feels. The Western physician uses an array of high-tech diagnostic equipment. In China, acupuncture and herbs are used extensively. By comparison, in the West, antibiotics and prescription drugs are used extensively. Both of these treatment modalities have enjoyed much success in spite of different origins and concepts. Antibiotics have overshadowed many effective treatments around the world for over fifty years. Unfortunately their use as a cure-all may be ending because of misuse. Antibiotics are becoming less effective. As a result, Western medicine may soon be put to a new test: how to effectively treat disease without antibiotics. Bacteria seem to have learned how to evolve with special immunity to antibiotics, especially when the antibiotics have been inappropriately used.

Ayurvedic medicine (a traditional Hindu system of treatments) is worthy of mention as another example of a philosophy and treatments that evolved before worldwide communication. According to Scott Gerson, M.D., this healing system dates back around 4,000 years to the Indus River Valley, an area now known as Pakistan. I find it revealing that Ayurvedic medicine has much in common, philosophically, with Chinese medicine. Both systems believe in life energy, i.e., Prana in the Ayurvedic system and (chi) in the Chinese system. It is more than a spark that animates living creatures! I agree with their philosophies that it is a far-reaching cosmic consciousness (God, if you prefer) that connects everything in the universe.

Without going into the detail about the seven Dhatus, the three Malas, and the three Doshas—Vata, Pitta, and Kapha and their respective breakdowns, I see a commonality between philosophies that didn't come from some sort of cultural exchange. Without communication or means of comparison these separate cultures (Ayurvedic and Chinese) developed effective treatments and uses for local herbs. Could it be that God provided, from the beginning, all that was needed to live a full and healthy life within any given culture? If so, what's missing? I think it has always been our lack of obedience and a distorted quest for truth. If properly sought, herbs, energy, spirituality, self control, proper physical activity and diet have always been available to mankind in every culture.

In the New Age Holistic Directory there are 140 listings of healing practices in the United States which are indexed to 175 pages of practitioners. The list does not include any standard American medical practices. My purpose in mentioning this bit of trivia is to show the availability of many treatment modalities in our own country. It would benefit us all to know a lot about these modalities. We should know as much about other treatment modalities as we do about American treatments. Knowing about what's available has saved my life twice. Consequently, I cannot resist promoting personal knowledge and choice.

Now that we are well into the Information Age, keeping up may seem harder to do. True, there is much advancement in many areas. However, technology actually makes it easier to keep up than ever before. Histories and current events are available at the touch of a button. Massive research and evaluation can now take place in hours, weeks or months that were impossible just a few years ago. To wit, the recent completion of mapping the human genetic code, a scientific advance that will take us to new dimensions of understanding, perhaps some not even expected as yet. As knowledge expands it helps us come closer to full understanding but it never should be allowed to invalidate existing knowledge. At this time the greatest threat to effective medicine is losing direction and purpose.

Are we ever going to be allowed to achieve all knowledge? I think not! Assuming God created it all, He must be the only power that is omnipotent and omniscient. As mortals, we are burdened by the dimensions of time and matter, matter consisting of materials of our own earth. There must be power that exists without matter, or possibly matter existing beyond our abilities of perception.

Everything mentioned in this article covers a wide range of ideas and treatments, all spawned by efforts to identify healing methods. But the purpose of this article is to identify the Master Healer. I defy anyone to come up with a simple and complete definition. However, I feel I have come close to identifying it by participating in my own healing of heart disease, rheumatoid arthritis, Sjogren's syndrome and cancer (lymphoma). I have acquired a partial understanding of the Master Healer through personal experience and study. However, I am convinced that complete understanding is unlikely in our time. What is it?

The Master Healer is a **PROCESS** within the brain that is active at all times. It is affected by everything we do. Each individual can learn about it and can control it. It is an element of each individual's makeup and, of course, we are all similar but different. It is obviously not simple or easy.

This **PROCESS** within the brain is a constant effort to achieve and maintain the balance we need for optimum healthy existence. Constant change and variation within and outside the body requires this process to be unique to each individual. It is continuous and it seldom, if ever, achieves a point of perfect balance.

All the various healing philosophies and treatment modalities were developed because of efforts to identify the nature of healing and establish treatments that would affect the process in a positive way. From the beginning, limited success has evolved by trial, error and experimentation. New technology should reduce these difficulties but it will not fully identify or explain some of the components of the **PROCESS**.

One of the most complicating aspects of this **PROCESS** is a person's denial of his own role, or a failure to recognize that the ability to fully heal lies within himself. All the healing efforts put forth by doctors and all the health aids of drugs and good diet only influence what goes on within the individual. A doctor can repair a broken bone or administer a very effective drug which may bring about recovery. However, elements of the "healing brain" must be properly involved or the patient will perish.

I call the brain "healing" because it manages all involuntary processes and influences all voluntary processes as well. If the patient is aware of his own healing capacities he can greatly influence the **PROCESS**. Sometimes the patient can command the **PROCESS** and effect healing without any help or interference.

I have personally found it possible to cross that barrier which separates conscious activity from the subconscious. This ability can be acquired by anyone. It must be a very personalized thing for each individual. I learned how to control a number of things that go on in my body that are obvious and other things that are obscure to the senses. They are controlled by the brain and a form of cellular intelligence.

The next few paragraphs are about personal experience with cancer and what I learned while establishing my own treatment program. It was April of 1991 and I was in serious trouble. I had just been diagnosed with cancer.

I had, for many years, used mostly natural healing methods for a variety of lesser ailments. I also used a good medical doctor for diagnostics and some drug prescriptions. I still do. I suppose I differ from the norm, being very critical of most recommended treatments. The more the patient knows about healing, the more likely he will be healed.

After discovering lumps in my stomach, first by personal examination, then CAT scans followed by exploratory surgery, I was informed that I had cancer. It was a plus stage three small cell lymphoma which had metastasized. There was one large tumor in the mesentery of the stomach and six smaller tumors in the liver. There was absolutely no questions about the diagnosis, still a part of hospital records. I was immediately given a prognosis by the resident oncologist. He didn't suggest, he directed me to begin chemotherapy and radiation as soon as I could leave the hospital, with the comment that I could only expect to live six months if I did not follow his explicit instructions. He seemed very anxious to begin treatment and more concerned about his advanced fee than he was about my health. I would not submit to chemotherapy and I had no other immediate plan. This was a difficult and lonely moment in my life. Contrary to the oncologist's expressed belief, I knew I had time to organize my thoughts and decide on a course of treatment.

Cancer is a cellular disorder. I knew that chemotherapy and radiation both had dangerous side effects, most notably the destruction of cells, both good and bad. Since I already had cellular destruction caused by the cancer, more cellular destruction made about as much sense as a rubber crutch! I needed a program that would repair and heal cells.

I set out to design such a program in spite of much advice to the contrary. The oncologist actually pestered me with his warnings and my family had already been convinced to encourage me to accept his treatment. In my mind it was a shortcut to death. What did I learn from this? Don't submit to a procedure you do not believe in. You then have no control and it probably will not work.

Assuming that we are all tested in this life, this was my supreme test. I knew a little about meditation and mind control. I knew about herbs, vitamins and diet and used them for lesser ailments. I did not know how to put my program together. I got some good naturopathic advice, studied a lot and did a lot of self experimentation. I did not know what it would eventually include. It was very dynamic for the first three years. And even now, after ten years and a complete remission, I doubt this healing program has ever been duplicated, before or since. And it should only be duplicated in a general way because each such program needs to be personalized.

I had to know that each element of the treatment would be OK for me. It was a matter between me, my healing brain, my cellular condition and my body in general. The Healing Brain Process will not respond in a positive manner unless you know your actions will encourage healing. Anything contrary to this will cause harm.

I was able to develop an approach to meditation just for my situation. To do so I studied Reiki (an ancient healing technique using energy transfer), transcendental meditation, relaxation meditation, visualization techniques, and prayer. To achieve benefits from my technique required study and practice. In the next few paragraphs, I will explain how I put my program together.

For greater detail, see the chapter on developing your own program.

Most people using transcendental meditation require the use of a mantra as a means of directing focus. My focus was directed to my illness. I studied the cellular nature, chemistry and all things known to affect the illness. I then applied relaxation therapy to put myself in a state of complete relaxation, isolating me from all distraction. At this point I used an effective form of visualization which made it possible for me to project myself into any given body function. In this program, my goal was to command cellular behavior. I felt I was able to command the production of new cells from the zygote stage (the original 46 chromosome cell) to mitosis multiplication (constant formation of new cells). I was also able to direct the process of differentiation (assignment of new cells to various parts of the body) to defective parts of the body requiring new cells for fortification and recovery. During this process I was able to increase formation of new killer "T" cells, interferon and macrophage activity. I used prayer at the beginning and at the end of this exercise to put myself at one with the powers of deity asking for permission, approval and success. These activities are usually automatic brain functions. And, of course, cellular intelligence is deep and somewhat remote to our conscious mind. Even the research biologists cannot identify the mechanism of differentiation (that which directs one cell to develop the eye and another to develop the toenail). We all know it happens, we just don't know how. But, I now know that automatic functions of the brain can be influenced by an individual's active mind.

After two years, I was cancer free. It has now been ten years and I feel reasonably safe in proclaiming success in my ability to identify and use my Master Healer.

Do mind control and cellular intelligence seem a bit far out, maybe a bit out of reach? It may seem that way but it's not so. These and a few other "far out" things constitute the real healing process.

The following terms denote what I am talking about. Unfortunately they are often used interchangeably, and incorrectly: meditation, mind, self, spirit and soul. These terms represent keys to healing even though few people understand them in that context. Another group of more common terms is equally important to healing: attitudes, beliefs, expectations, faith, feelings, perceptions, society, deity and prayer. Still three more here that have special meaning to anyone in the healing business: mind control, placebo and spiritual healing.

It is easier to understand the efficacy of some situations by merely looking at what happens and then thinking it out. A few common examples: A medical doctor examines a person very carefully then tells him with some disdain, "Go home, it's all in your head." The doctor doesn't realize the person is already sick, before his testing can detect any problem.

Sometimes a doctor cannot see all that goes on in the many complexities that control the body. The patient goes home angry. He knows something is wrong. He will probably go home and suffer until the disease progresses to an obvious stage, maybe too late for help. A better option is not to wait but go to a doctor that practices naturopathy, uses kinesiology, herbs, enzymes and vitamins. The naturopathic doctor may be able to help bring the patient's body into balance and quick recovery.

Beliefs—have you ever seen a seriously ill person get well when he believed he would not recover? A man's beliefs can be a reflection of how he is using his Master Healer.

Faith—on the other hand, the person above may experience a complete recovery if he cultivates a positive attitude and has faith in his own ability to heal.

We all know that mind, sense of self, spirit, and soul are strong determinants of every aspect of our existence.

Mind Control—can be evidenced by the power of WILL in addition to aspects explained in my own story.

Placebo Effect—is evident in many forms. If a person believes it, so it will be. Volumes have been written about this one healing feature, a feature totally controlled by some unknown brain function. The placebo effect is so firm and dependable that medical science uses it as a basis for testing most new drugs, i.e., the well-known double blind placebo tests. When a person is given an inert pill (sugar or even colored water) it will cause healing at a fairly reliable level, provided that person believes he is getting the real drug. When a new drug is introduced, a double blind study is one of the FDA requirements for approval. All the pills are made to appear alike. Half of the test participants get the placebo and half actually get the new drug. If the new drug gets better results, even by a small margin, the new drug will usually be approved and applauded as successful. This is a good example of brain involvement in the healing process. So far, the mechanics of this phenomenon is not understood.

Spiritual Healing—can take place in many ways. The most frequently seen by me is the healing that takes place under the direction of priestly authority and usually involves laying on of hands. Some people are healed by going to places designated as "holy." Lourdes in France, though controversial, receives thousands of visitors every year seeking spiritual healing.

Prayer—is a controversial and mysterious process that has been with us since the beginning. NEWSWEEK, March 31, 1997, published an opinion poll: 87% of participants say that God answers prayers, 82% say they ask for health or success, 79% say God answers prayers for healing someone with an incurable disease.

Several hospital surveys have shown that patients prayed for had better recovery rates than those not prayed for.

This is a fascinating subject that touches every part of our existence. Your knowledge will save your life. My objective here is to provide enough information to prove there is a Master Healer. The brain is its control center. Everyone has a Master Healer. All should learn to use it. There are many approaches to healing besides standard American medicine. Choose carefully. Many American doctors are great helpers in the healing process. Some are uncaring licensed drug dealers. Choose your doctor wisely.

For those interested in exploring related subjects. I recommend the following for reference and interesting reading:

Ageless Body Timeless Mind (et al)

Deepak Chopra,MD

Harmony Books

Spontaneous Healing (et al)

Andrew Weil, MD

Ballantine Books

Love, Medicine & Miracles

Bernie S. Siegel, MD

Harper & Row Publishers

The Healing Brain

Robert Ornstein, Phd

and

David Sobel, MD

Simon & Schuster

The Three-Pound Universe

Judith Hooper

and

Dick Teresi

Macmillan Publishing

PART III: AVAILABLE HEALTH TREATMENTS - GETTING THE JOB DONE

The preceding parts of this book have emphasized various philosophies and problems within the American system of health treatment. I have repeatedly told my own story, or parts of it, to emphasize the gravity of the health problems involved and the fact that the information in this book came from my own personal experience and study. Today's research efforts are directed in a manner that offers major rewards for promising pharmaceutical solutions to disease. It seems more logical to me if much more research were directed toward healing and strengthening the immune system thereby allowing the body to heal itself naturally. I am convinced that self healing is the only true healing and that the body was designed to function in a normal manner. Perhaps the pharmaceutical solution is the reason why we have so many systemic disorders that result in long-term illnesses. I am convinced that the answer is fairly simple. It involves things we do to our own bodies and to the environment which interfere with the basic intended functions of the body. If a person has a diagnosis of a systemic disease, especially cancer, and if the prognosis involves at least a few months to live, I believe one can heal himself. In fact, I know one can heal himself because I have done it.

Is cancer curable? I know it is! However, the trick is to know and understand the "many" alternative treatments and to establish a treatment plan that will work for the person who has such a disorder. The next few chapters will be helpful in showing how this may be done. They include many products used in my own plan as well as a number of natural products that are often referred to as alternative treatments.

In my case, I had no direction in the beginning, no starting point and no routine. I sort of "felt my way along" because I had no experience and little room for mistakes. This worked for me because I am sensitive to what goes on in my body, I am curious, and I try very hard to get answers and to do what I think is right.

It pays to be attentive and cautious. It seems that each doctor, teacher, researcher, or peddler pushes his or her own product as if it were the only answer. One thing I have found out for sure, no one person has the complete answer. Real truth sometimes lies in combinations of available techniques. My personal experience has found this to be true. I rely a lot on standard American medicine for diagnostics and I use some prescription drugs for things I am sure about. For everything else, I rely on Naturopathic doctors and natural products as noted in some of the chapters in this part of the book.

Probably the most crippling thing in the medical group's search for cures is this very situation where each party will not venture away from their own technique or culture. This is especially true when pharmaceutical research is involved. These companies are bound by the dollar, to only serve the project that brings in the bucks. Much wrong doing comes from this situation.

The chapters in Part III will list various products, procedures, and life styles which will affect healing and health in general. These chapters include items I know about first hand. The list includes alternatives to the standard medical fare of chemotherapy and radiation. I exclude detailed discussion of standard medical treatments here because they are usually self serving, well advertised, well known and there are many volumes (pro and con) on this subject.

So far, there have been few satisfactory answers coming from the establishment, therefore, many people are looking for their own answers. I am a living example that they are doing this with considerable success.

Morris "J" Llewellyn

CHAPTER 8: THE SIX DIMENSIONS OF HEALTH

The six dimensions of health are also the six dimensions of illness. We often hear one of these factors referred to individually but I don't recall ever hearing them referred to as a group. In establishing a healing program for myself, I think of these six things as guidelines for diagnostic analysis. I try to honestly evaluate each item one at a time. I do this in an attempt to establish a baseline profile for my original analysis. I repeat this periodically as an evaluative tool for my own progress. These items are listed below. The comments are intended to help me gain insight.

1. SPIRITUAL - This is one of those terms mentioned in chapter 7 that's poorly defined in places like the dictionary. At least part of such a definition must come from our own spiritual nature, and it is different for each individual. The spiritual nature of things, and the definition of spiritual, will be influenced by one's religion, philosophy and relationships with people and with Deity; and rightfully so. For the purpose of this personal analysis, I need to feel good, or at least acceptable, toward the spiritual elements of my life. If there is anything wrong here I must correct it before I can effectively use my energies toward healing.

2. PSYCHOLOGICAL/MENTAL - Sometimes these elements blend with the spiritual. The part that separates the mental from the spiritual is

dimensional. Spiritual is personal and not firmly defined by our peers. Whereas, psychological and mental are pretty firmly defined by medical authority and strongly influenced by peer judgements. Psychological and mental elements clearly affect physical health. And environmental situations can strongly affect mental health. Care should be exercised if there is any question about psychosis or neurosis.

My personal opinion is that too many shrinks are themselves unstable and are looking for easy money via long term analysis. Conversely, short term analysis can be very effective when conducted by a good professional. If you find that you have a real problem in this area, it should be resolved as soon as possible. It is difficult to be effective with your own efforts in natural physical healing if there is any psychological impediment.

3. NUTRITIONAL - Most poor health in the world is related to life style. Aside from exercise, diet is the single most dominant factor in health. In this country, we usually eat every day, and we do it from birth until we depart from this existence. The hungry children in Africa to opulent fatties in the United States represent the scope and breadth of this problem. Some don't get enough to eat and others do little else (other than eating)!

To be successful in your own natural healing program you must have reasonable nutritional health. If your primary problem is nutritional, see chapter nine on DIETARY HABITS.

4. PHYSICAL/CHEMICAL - The organs, primarily liver, kidneys and adrenal glands, serve as the body's own chemical factory. A normal healthy body can produce precise amounts of chemicals and hormones as needed under circumstances that, at times, change in an instant. No external mechanism can do this.

Medical technology attempts to supplement this function with drugs when some part of the body fails and needs help. This is done with varying degrees of success. Before attempting a self healing program, an understanding of any currently used drug program is necessary. What are the drugs involved? What do they do? Can they impact the effect of a proposed natural healing program? Feel comfortable and assured that the elements of your healing program do not conflict.

Proper physical factors can be a very large factor in health and current condition. A body properly cared for will diminish the need for externally administered drugs. Such proper care is usually very simple consisting of appropriate amounts of exercise and rest.

5. GENETIC - Genetic factors sometimes strongly affect health. Understand any existing genetic factors that may influence health in your family. Knowing of such factors usually gives a person warnings and the ability to compensate. Great success has been realized compensating for genetic problems using natural healing techniques. In establishing a healing

program feel right about such factors. Know what the compensating things are, usually diet, exercise, and supplements.

6. PURPOSE - Having purpose in life provides a magical healing factor that seems to be totally irreplaceable. This seems to be a very strong psychological element in healing and in attaining old age. Several studies have shown that people, even with long term ailments, tend to survive to 100 years and beyond when they have purpose. What is worthwhile purpose? To an observer it may seem trivial. To the subject it is something that demands attention, something that must be done, something that demands living for. It can be as simple as seeing a pet through its life span. Most of the cases I have read about involve a feeling of being needed or wanting to see a task come to fruition. If you want to feel good about living for a long time, involve yourself in something you see as an essential activity. My wife's special purpose in life is to record the life histories of each of our grandchildren. The task becomes larger with each birth. I know she has no plans to stop this activity. Maybe she will set a new record for attaining old age.

CHAPTER 9: DIETARY HABITS

For the most part our "bad" dietary habits produce two things, poor health and feces! Is this statement extreme? I don't think so. In a country of plenty, in a country of high technology, we should be able to do wonderful things with diet. Actually we are able, but for the most part we do not. The public is not concerned enough until it is too late. And the profit motive rules how information is given to the public.

For those who are seriously interested, there are many approaches to establishing a good diet. Hucksters by the thousands are attempting to sell plans and products at just about every turn. Obviously, selecting a helpful plan in this environment is very difficult. The two dominant positions on diet have been taken by two well trained doctors: Robert C. Atkins, M.D. and John A. McDougall, M.D.

These doctors are well established respected authorities on the various effects of diet on health. The interesting thing about this is that each doctor approaches the effects of diet on health as paramount, but they oppose each other's approach vigorously. Their debates have been published and televised widely. Obviously they cannot both be right on every issue. Thousands of other "diet experts" have taken similar polarized positions.

Establishing a dietary plan using this large body of information is next to impossible.

There is too much advice and technical guidance in the many books published by these two doctors. Dr. Atkins is a great supporter of heavy use of proteins and very little use of carbohydrates. Whereas, Dr. McDougall's approach is almost the reverse making heavy use of carbohydrates and very light use of proteins such as meats and animal fats. I find the writings of both of these doctors interesting and well done. I cannot strongly support or reject either position. The thing I find difficult and damaging for simple folk such as myself is that I am overwhelmed by so much expert advice (some of it in conflict) that I am unable to effectively use it.

I see a serious need for simple solutions for people trying to establish good health practices. Many of us get bogged down in too much expert dietary advice. So, I give you my simple solution, use some of the old fashioned expert advice that came from grandma's kitchen. These were her rules which seemed to work very nicely: (1) Be sure to keep caloric intake in balance with energy needs. This wasn't difficult when we worked long days in the fields. Hunger dictated the need for food. (2) Every meal was timed and each meal consisted of fresh protein such as eggs or meat, whole wheat home baked bread, at least two fruits or vegetables, and desert at lunch and dinner. Plenty of good water was always available. Meals were peaceful and orderly, usually preceded by prayers of thanks. For those who were still hungry there was plenty of fruit and other farm produce.

I don't remember any fat or sickly people in the family back then. The key had to be a good balance between food intake, exercise, rest and possibly good spring water. Exercise equated to long days of hard labor on the farm. A few hours a week at one of the few exercise facilities was strictly for entertainment, such as basketball or boxing. In present culture, being faced by a hard day of physical work is almost rare. Being over fed and under worked is currently a major threat to basic health.

In grandma's time I didn't know a protein from a carbohydrate, I never ate anything from a box or a can with the possible exception of salt, sugar and some cereals. I never heard of store bought vitamins, minerals, or prepared foods. Well, for my lazy self, thank goodness those days are over. Modern convenience is great, but what has it done to us? We tend to eat crap endlessly: ready made meals (fast foods of all kinds). Practically everything is partly prepared and in a can or a box which means it has been preserved with some combination of chemicals.

People seem to be too lazy to buy fresh produce or even read labels to determine what's going into the body. Wow! No wonder our over-fed and under-exercised kids are becoming obese and diabetic! Lets not forget the effect of fast foods with the extra salt, the excess calories and the poisonous effect of the excess fats that become trans-fatty acids in deep fried cooking. It now becomes evident why many of us adults follow the easy path and end up with long term illnesses in our latter years.

Now, if this advice and grandma's methods don't do it for you, and you sense illness, go to a good gastroenterologist. They specialize in knowing all about stomach function and stomach disease.

I see most of us having some trouble with the diet and exercise thing. The busy world we live in today makes it difficult to properly care for ourselves when it comes to diet and exercise. This very situation has made it necessary to add chapter 10 on the use of nutritional supplements and exercise as a basic part of a good health plan.

Grandma's kitchen served good food as well as setting a good example. However, I know most of us rely on other sources of advice for more up-to-date guidance, something more appropriate for our time. I have some of that too. Our objective is to set a simple course for achieving and maintaining good health. A good simple diet is absolutely essential to achieve this goal.

As noted in the early chapters, I have been burdened by some very harsh disorders. I have elected to design my own treatments and diets. I don't suggest that others go quite this far. But if you want to survive long-term, know what you are doing and why you are doing it.

With thousands of dietary books out there offering meal by meal plans, scientific analysis of meals, projecting a variety of results for the old, and the vital adult, you already have a problem of complexity. Then, of course, most of these costly plans are obligated to give lengthy projections of results on almost everything, nice skin, youthfulness, weight loss, regaining sexual abilities of youth, and almost anything else you desire. So complicated that few people who buy the plans are able to live by them.

And what's to worry about, you already have an automatic planning and distribution system that beats them all. It's called your body. It's simple and it's easy! Admittedly you must accept some control to make it work well. But it will.

For those who are seriously ill, some special medical help may be needed. But for the most part your own body will figure out how much it wants and what to do with it. Some selective control is necessary. The body is like a computer or a fine machine, garbage in, garbage out. Good fuel will produce good clean energy. Foods don't need to be modified to provide good input.

Two things essential to a good diet: natural input and simple preparation.

Use whole grain cereals and breads. Too much processing is not good for any foods. Use lots of vegetables, both cooked and raw. Also use lots of fresh fruits. Only apples seem to be appropriate for mixing with vegetables at the same time. Use seeds and nuts in moderation. How about desert? Be careful with sugar. Dark chocolate in moderation agrees with me and is supported by some of the "experts". I think it is good to decide for yourself on some controversial items. I like the boost given by coffee but apparently the caffeine is all it has to offer. Tea, especially green tea, can give a smaller shot of caffeine but has much more to offer in the way of good health. It has great antioxidant qualities.

As for safe preparation, don't use aluminum cook ware. Cast iron or glass is better. I recommend using a juicer because of freshness and high concentration of nutritional values per volume. There are several people who are adamant about the health and healing values of juicing. It is easy to locate good juice machines on the market. I use juicing products sold by Stephen Sinatra, M.D. and Jay Kordich (the juiceman) because they have good machines and many good juicing recipes in their literature. Their products are especially good for those who are interested in juicing for special health issues such as weight loss and specific ailments.

Cooking with complex recipes can be troublesome for some people. Complex recipes also introduce too many questionable additives, and unhealthy oils. The best way is to keep it simple. I do Japanese style hibachi with a cast iron skillet and very light cooking oil such as Canola or

PAM. Olive oil is best but don't get it too hot. Steam cooking and cooking bags work well. Use things that are easy and items that you don't mind doing repeatedly.

I think my approach is the best way to go. It has worked very well for me. Start as simple as possible. Then add carefully as you learn what is right for you. I have used this approach in every element of my health activity. Diet is paramount but I have used the same technique when selecting supplements, herbal medications, natural treatments, exercise routines and even medical treatments. Along with this approach, I have selected a medical doctor that is open to the use of any natural methods that work. This doctor is the one I use for diagnostic testing. This medical doctor knows about the health treatments I use and the success I have had.

When starting a new diet keep it simple and use some of your favorite foods. Eat what makes you happy as long as it also makes you well. There is so much good stuff out there that this is possible. A good diet should become a part of your long term life style. Be comfortable with new diet changes, then it will be easy to eliminate items that need to be eliminated.

I use many books for reference purposes, for general education and for gleaning dietary and health tidbits. I recommend this technique but if one is not highly selective it can waste a lot of time. I have read hundreds of books in an effort to find the best sources of dietary and natural healing information. Exhaustive research has always brought me back to solutions similar to the ones I learned in grandma's kitchen.

There are some old ailments that have recently proliferated in our society which require some special dietary adjustments. I have been my own guinea pig in selecting the correct mix of supplements and items to be eliminated or added to a good diet plan. An appropriate example is diabetes. In this difficult case we need to pay attention to the glucose food index when evaluating the items in diets for diabetics.

Diet is one of the main avenues of control over diabetes. A good version of the glycemic index is listed on the internet at http://www.mendosa.com/gilists.htm. I have elected not to repeat this list in its entirety because it is a list of raw numbers and it is 22 pages long. This same site offers a great deal of information on diabetes. Start your own diet incorporating foods that are organically grown, fresh and simply prepared. If possible, meats should be range grown and fully cooked. I list only a few foods here that are good for stable blood sugar: apples, artichokes, asparagus, beet greens, broccoli, brown rice, cauliflower, celery, chicken, chicory, cranberries, endive, fava beans, kidney beans, fish, garlic, grapefruit, leaf lettuce, lemons, lima beans, millet, olives and olive oil, onions, peppers, seeds and nuts in small quantities, and turkey. Start your own diet with simple preparations and add to your diet and other aspects of your program by reviewing the reference data. Reference data has been simplified by my efforts to list a few good sources from hundreds of books. You will add other good sources as you develop your own program.

The following books are offered as references. They are appropriate additions to the things talked about in this book. They contain a lot of specific dietary information that applies to almost every health condition.

NATURAL TREATMENTS FOR DIABETES

By Kathi Head, N.D.—Prima Publishing

EARL MINDELL'S FOOD AS MEDICINE

By Earl Mindell, R. Ph., Ph.D.—Fireside of Simon & Schuster

FOOD—YOUR MIRACLE MEDICINE

By Jean Carper—Harper Collins Publishers, Inc.

The above books are good for spot reference or extensive study. These authors are trained and competent researchers in this field. Their purpose is not to sell a product but to provide good information to their readers.

When illnesses require dietary adjustments for medical reasons be careful and consult with your doctor.

Morris "J" Llewellyn

CHAPTER 10: NUTRITIONAL

SUPPLEMENTATION AND EXERCISE

Diet, Supplementation, and Exercise are the troika of natural health and healing. Attention to these areas will provide all the help most people need.

If the perfect person (which I haven't met yet) were born and raised in good health and had a proper plan and gave it full participation he would be healthy and could live to be 120 years old. Its too bad that so many people die unnecessarily young, especially between the ages of 55 and 75. Causes of death are numerous according to medically issued death certificates. In my opinion, the base cause of death in this group is ignorance and disinterest in the subject of good health and long life. Disease, even death, can be delayed with proper natural treatments.

This also applies to genetic disorders. It is not hard to compensate for some genetic weaknesses. Cardiac function is a prime example. If a person knows about tendencies toward heart dysfunction in his family he can sometimes live a long and full life by merely following sensible diet, supplementation and exercise. After evaluation, adding extra vitamin E, COQ-10, and magnesium may extend his life considerably. On the other hand, a person who looks good, feels good, and performs well may experience sudden death after a few years of neglecting these same precautions.

Some of my medical friends will come down hard on me for being so adamant about natural healing. However, I have discussed this at length with some of them, and if I personalize the discussion, most of them agree with the things I say, especially the content of this chapter. The only argument I can get for not participating in programs to improve and lengthen life is, and I quote, "I am trained to treat illness with drugs and surgery and that's all I do". I think that is the most honest answer I ever received from a medical doctor.

Most of us need a basic nutritional supplement program and a moderate exercise program to go with our sensible diet. As with diet, we get a tremendous amount of over complication caused by our own interest in all kinds of supplementation. There's also a huge and profitable market out there anxious to satisfy our every desire and curiosity. Unfortunately the suppliers are too numerous and poorly regulated. To reap the many benefits available from supplementation, we need to be cautious and well informed about the products we buy.

So, in this complex environment, how does one establish a good supplementation program? To work well, the elements of simplicity used in other programs must be included in this program.

This is how I did mine.

To start, I accept the premise that we all need a base program that provides the basic requirements of vitamins and minerals. There are a number of suppliers that provide good products for this need either in the form of made up packages for daily use or a specified number of tablets each day from a bottle. These are designed to provide total basic daily requirements. I have used at least five suppliers over time and found them to all be at least acceptable. These products were all designed by reliable doctors. My only caution, as usual, always read labels for all the products you use. Over time you will become very knowledgeable about the products you use and which ones are best for you.

I stress the fact that this is a good place to start for everybody. Because of our modern day environment we all need basic supplementation.

As a young adult this approach helped me and gave me a boost. Typically, as I got older I saw the need for various other supplements. This is when one needs to exercise some expertise and care. All the peddlers have a "special product" for every ailment and condition known to man. I suppose this is good if you can "sort the wheat from the chaff". Over time, I have learned how to do this.

As noted earlier in the book, I have a fairly large number of ongoing ailments. For most of my treatments I self prescribe natural products. I can do this because of years of study and self experimentation. I now know what works for me. For us all, it isn't necessary to rush into using new products. In fact, be very cautious! Unproven prescription drugs and "new" natural products often fall short of original hype.

I have suppliers that provide a great deal of information on the products they sell. This helps to simplify my problem of keeping track of what I am doing and why. As noted above, I have changed my base program several times to accommodate what I want to do with my total supplement program.

I had a heart problem several years ago and I now have to add another problem, I am diabetic. For this reason I want my base of daily vitamins and minerals to be lighter (definitely not in the megadose range) allowing me to add natural health treatments to my daily routine without overloading.

To help you establish good sources of natural products, I am listing four places I have done business with. They have all given me prompt service and good products. It has been easier for me to assemble a basic program of compatible products from a single supplier. However, I use the listed references for many special products designed and controlled by doctors who have expanded their knowledge to cover natural healing methods and products. They all provide good product information and they all offer monthly news/research papers free or for a very reasonable price.

*****STEPHEN SINATRA, M.D.

A Fellow of the American College of Cardiology;

Fellow of the American College of Nutrition;

board certified in internal medicine and cardiology;

certified in anti-aging medicine, clinical nutrition and

bioenergetic analysis.

This doctor offers a full line of supplements including a basic supplement program (DAILY NUTRIENT PROGRAM} and a catalog of other compatible advanced supplements. He also has a monthly report (the Sinatra Health Report). This doctor currently provides my basic daily program and compatible cardiac supplements. Additional information and ordering at drsinatra.com and free calls at 1-800-304-1708.

*****JULIAN WHITAKER, M.D.

FOUNDER & DIRECTOR OF WHITAKER WELLNESS INSTITUTE

AUTHOR OF DR. WHITAKER'S GUIDE TO NATURAL HEALING

AUTHOR AND PUBLISHER OF HEALTH & HEALING NEWSLETTER

This doctor offers a full line of supplements. His basic formula (THE FORWARD PLUS REGIMEN) is full strength and includes 42 nutrients in

2 packets per day. Additional product information usually accompanies each product order. The wellness institute can provide professional assistance in designing programs for treating various ailments. When adding to basic programs, pay attention to product compatibility and total amounts taken. Additional information and ordering at drwhitaker.com and free calls at 1-800-722-8008.

*****DR. DAVID WILLIAMS

FOUNDER & EDITOR OF "ALTERNATIVES", A MONTHLY JOURNAL OF ALTERNATIVE MEDICINE.

This doctor is well known for his research of alternative health treatments on a world wide basis. Much of his research has resulted in the introduction of new health treatments from around the world, especially from Australia. He offers a baseline vitamin and mineral package under the name of "Daily Advantage, Multi-Nutrient System". Many other natural treatments are available with attendant educational literature. Additional information and ordering at DrDavidWilliams.com. Supplement orders at 1-800-304-1708 and publications at 1-800-843-8408.

*****NATURE'S DISTRIBUTORS, INC., presents "THE HEALTHY CELL NEWS". MICHAEL MINARSICH, PRESIDENT AND DR. DECKER WEISS RESIDENT DOCTOR AND PRODUCT DESIGNER.

This publication's success is marked by seventeen years of publication. Free to all customers. It's purpose is to promote "The Healthy Cell Concept" as a part of healthy living by offering natural health products in each monthly issue. Each issue also publishes very good data on the products they sell as well as special articles about the healthy cell concept.

Four easy ways to order: 1-800-624-7114, 24 hours per day, 7 days per week. Secure web site www.naturesdistributors.com. Fax 1-480-837-8420. Mail order address: Nature's Distributors, Inc. 16508 E. Laser Dr., Bldg. B, Fountain Hills, AZ 85268.

Thousands of suppliers exist out there and I am sure many of them are Ok. This list of suppliers is intended to simplify your job of putting together a good simple nutritional program that can be easily maintained.

This chapter includes exercise, the third item of the natural healing Troika.

I find it amusing when surfing the internet to note the many avenues of study one can follow in these three areas of human fitness. Good diet is a must, good nutrient supplementation is critical, and appropriate exercise is essential for life. While the technical aspects of study in these areas reach high levels, the basics are simple and easily realized by the average individual. So why are so many people sick and dependent? My opinion doesn't cost anything and it doesn't come from medical training but here it is anyway.

At the first sign of pain or dysfunction many people want someone else to give them the magic touch or the cure all pill that will extend youth and vitality. That's unrealistic. On this level no such help exists. No such help will ever exist.

The bodies we are given are amazingly strong, self maintained and self healing. However we are the intelligence that directs and cares for the body. We must at least give it care and maintenance to enjoy its durability and longevity of somewhere between 80 and 120 years. We have already talked about diet and supplementation. Exercise remains to be examined. I see it as the most vital of all long term elements of good health. It is so easy to succumb to the urge to relax that it sometimes becomes the primary thing we do. TV, elevators, escalators, one story ramblers, golf carts and the list goes on and on that identifies our energy saving devices. If we don't use a little energy now and then, the body will die. This is very contrary to our nature. God gave us the mechanism to at least run for protection and survival if need be. It isn't hard to maintain that much energy.

I asked a doctor friend the simplest answer to this problem. He snapped back with a very direct answer: "get off your dead butt and do something, move around a lot. Watch the little kids at play, you'll get the idea". This was his practical advice for the under active adult. This guy speaks from experience. He is a medical doctor with specialties in cardiology, atomic medicine and sports medicine. I do not mean to underplay the importance of advanced study in these areas. What I do mean to do is emphasize the importance of simple activity to basic health. While some extensive exercise plans can stimulate special benefits, total inactivity can be fatal.

Many areas of study in each of these areas reach the level of doctorate degrees and beyond into many areas of research. Advanced exercise plans can promote great strength and superb conditioning which are not usually needed for good health. Yet many individuals tend to come up short by ignoring the major benefit of simple exercise to their health and longevity. Even more amusing is the fact that life saving knowledge in these areas is available to all at practically no cost. No training necessary even for the likes of me.

For the purpose of this message, it is clear and simple, just do something! For those interested in professional training programs and higher education, one needs only to go to "exercise or exercise physiology" on the internet. In looking for further information, I found two very effective approaches, (1) use the search engine GOOGLE or go directly to htt://www.acefitness.org.

For a simple at home gym that works wonders for shut-ins and others that have limited mobility, one only needs the following items. A small amount of motivation can produce remarkable results and maintain good conditioning.

A small roll-up mat.

An exercise rebounder (a very low impact trampoline).

A treadmill.

A few dumbbells ranging from 2 to 35 lbs.

To your everlasting health, exercise and keep moving.

CHAPTER 11: HOMEOPATHIC AND SPECIAL REMEDIES

Homeopathic remedies, and some special homemade remedies, have been very important in many of my treatment programs. Most medical doctors do not attempt treatment programs that involve these things. It may be because they don't know enough about them or because it's too dangerous and too much trouble to buck the directives of the AMA.

It's up to you to pursue treatments other than those promoted by the pharmaceutical companies. There are doctors who use treatments other than the ones promoted. Its good to know such a doctor before experiencing a health problem. Consult with that doctor before you use a treatment you are not familiar with.

Whenever I have a serious ailment and feel I need help, I make sure I get that kind of advice and consequently I use many treatments commonly used in other cultures. There are literally hundreds of approaches to healing, far too many to reiterate here. Dozens of reference texts are available that give detailed descriptions of these healing techniques. A reference library can be a powerful tool and should be used before consulting with any kind of doctor.

Many Ayurvedic medicines, Chinese medicines and homeopathic preparations have been around for a long time. Some of these treatments are effective even when our standard medical approach is not.

HOMEOPATHIC TREATMENTS are best explained by health professionals who use them. However there are only a few doctors who only practice homeopathy. Many doctors use homeopathic treatments such as naturopaths, chiropractors, and many medical doctors. Because of the financial, political, and practical considerations, some states require use of homeopathic and naturopathic treatments to be under the supervision of a medical doctor.

Homeopathy has been with us for a long time. A German chemist, Dr. Samuel Hahnemann is generally credited with the primary development of homeopathy in the early 1800's. With the resistance of organized medicine, the science has experienced many ups and downs but today over 2000 homeopathic remedies are in use. The science has had legal status in the United States since 1938. According to the National Center of Homeopathy in Alexandra, Va. there currently about 3000 recognized practitioners nationwide.

It is not just a passing fad nor is it an area of science without success. It is a method of medical treatment designed to stimulate the body's own healing processes. Homeopathy is based on the idea that likes are cured by likes. I.e., a substance that causes an illness can be used to cure that same illness if administered in very small doses that are prepared in a certain way. The process involves progressive testing and shaking. The process of healing seems to work in a way similar to immunization or the building up of an resistance to the substance that caused the illness. When the product comes to the ill person, treatment is as simple as administering a few drops under the tongue.

"When it works it can be dramatic. It seems as if a magical boost is given to the body's healing capacity." This quote is my own and I give it as a patient having first hand experience.

Homeopathy was widely practiced before antibiotics. Since the dominance of the AMA and the heavy influence of pharmaceutical interests, homeopathy almost became an abandoned science. As mentioned above, in recent years there has been a resurgence of its popularity paralleling the public demand for more naturopathic healing products and practices.

Most routine ailments are healed within a short time regardless of the approach used. I have often had the thought that patients get well in spite of treatment and that the natural healing abilities of the body are very much underrated by us all.

However, I have a standard rule that I think all serious patients should follow: "When receiving treatment for any disorder expect good results. If you don't get good results, if symptoms are not alleviated within a short period of time, say two visits, change your doctor." This is especially true for treatments that are supposed to give almost instantaneous results, such as, homeopathy, electric treatments, chiropractic, acupuncture, and drug treatments. There are many practitioners around for each specialty. Their experience and education levels vary a great deal. Don't entrust your life with someone you doubt.

If you are a "do it yourself" person like me, please note the following. Many special remedies have been developed over time as people have discovered the healing properties of various products. This has been going on since ancient times. Many of these products have been well proven and are in use today. They vary from the common things we come in contact with every day to exotic concoctions from jungle cultures. I have used many of these remedies with great success. You will find many remedies in your reference library, on the internet, and at your local health food store. For our purposes here, I can only review some good remedies and natural products with which I have used.

Just remember, know what you are doing. There is a long list of natural products that we all know. Some items are commonly known as foods but they have also been used in many ways as medicines and tonics in several cultures. Many of these common products are adaptogenic. Adaptogenic is a term used for products (primarily herbs) that have the ability to adapt to the body's health and healing needs. These products seem to be good for many things. To qualify for inclusion in this category the product must have no undesirable side effects. Not withstanding the fact that it is possible for any individual to be allergic to any given product.

Following are some of the "common" adaptogenic products I have used for my own ailments:

GINGER is one of the most widely used adaptogenic natural herbs in the world. It is a terrific food used in many ways. It is good with other vegetables as in stir fry. It is used in many ways as an additive spice. Most importantly, it is used in many ways as a medicinal treatment. One of the most common treatments, with which I am personally familiar, is for balance problems. It is more effective for sea sickness than many of the recommended drugs designed for dizziness. It is extremely effective in the treatment of morning sickness in pregnant women. Just a personal note about morning sickness: Our daughter was so troubled by morning sickness with her last pregnancy that many foods would not agree with her digestive system. Full strength ginger was one of them. The use of a light ginger ale gave her considerable relief. Ginger has been found to be very helpful in a variety of stomach ailments. It can be used in a variety of ways, raw, cooked, crystalized, and powdered extract in a capsule.

GARLIC is another very versatile product. It is widely used as a food which reportedly gives many benefits to users. It is one of the most effective natural antibiotics. It can stimulate cell growth and activity. It reportedly has very positive effects on human blood such as dissolving cholesterol, dilating blood vessels and reducing blood pressure.

OTHER ADAPTOGENIC HERBS include, but are not limited to, astragalus, Siberian ginseng, panax ginseng, shizandra, shitake, reishi and maitake mushrooms. If you are attempting to design your own cancer treatment program use of these products may be very helpful. I have used some of these products in pre-designed combinations. They are adaptogenic. Combinations are very useful and effective for some people and some conditions. However, if I were to use any combination, I would study and test using kinesiology techniques. I would then do some self experimentation. As I mentioned before, some people can be allergic to any product. I practice what I preach. I am very careful when I am unsure or when I do not know a given product well.

I want to continue with my list of very good products I have experienced or used. I do not want to assure the reader that the following herbs or remedies meet all the requirements of an adaptogenic, although some of them do. My list only includes some of the best I know. As you learn to research the products you use you will find the total list almost endless.

CAYENNE PEPPER is the most effective and versatile herb I have ever used in my own program. It can be obtained in several strengths and several forms. I use a great quantity of liquid extract for stimulating circulation and heart function. It is also available from herb shops as dried fruit, loose powder or in capsules.

I use a regular cayenne pepper extract and powders of about 45,000 heat units. It is available from approximately 20,000 to over 250,000 heat units. The red pepper family consists of many varieties. The pepper products used for health products come from African Bird Peppers, many Chinese and Asian varieties, Mexican Habaneros and California Jalapenos. Before using, check the heat units. Some varieties are very HOT! In addition to heart and circulation problems, these products are used for stomach problems including some ulcers, cream formulations are used for (arthritic) pain and skin disorders such as shingles.

COLLOIDAL SILVER is a fantastic product. I have used it since my cancer treatment days for many ailments. It is effective and there are no side effects.

Unfortunately there are some doctors who preach against its use. As yet I have found no good reason not to use it provided you know your product. Many times this is key to using a good product. There is always the chance that a product is adulterated by some unscrupulous producer, as can happen to any product that isn't controlled by law. Good labeling laws should be sufficient but the way around the occasional violator is to know your product well enough to recognize any flaw. Good quality is easy to recognize in Colloidal Silver. The following elements of good quality are easy to determine.

When properly made, colloidal silver, will remain in a very fine particle suspension. I.e., there will never be any particle sediment. The product will appear clear and clean even though it may have a slight amount of golden or amber color to it.

Manufacturing standards must include meticulous care in assuring perfection on three levels: Water purity, Particle Size, and Parts Per Million of silver.

Water must be very pure, distilled or revitalized ozonated water.

Particle size must be as small as possible. A good product can assure a particle size from 0.001 to 0.004 microns.

Parts per million (PPM) varies in accordance with strength preferred. 5 to 10 parts is effective for many internal disorders. I use 10 ppm for eyes and sinus. It has been very effective in my own treatment against pink eye and sinus infection providing an almost overnight cure. For stronger treatments of external and internal treatments I use 40 ppm. In some of my ailments it has been more effective than some of the new antibiotics.

Your local health food store will carry a line of colloidal minerals and pertinent data. Trimedica colloidal silver can be ordered by mail at 1-800-559-2873 or visit www.homecure,com. I also buy locally from Nature's Energy, Inc., 655 West 220 South, Suite 11, Pleasant Grove, UT 84062. Tel-785-2304

Follow the selection guidelines and a good product will not be hard to find. Dosage recommendations will be given on the label.

ALOE VERA is a very good skin treatment and is good for minor infections and burns (including sunburn). It is good for many external problems and is promoted by some health product manufactures for some internal uses such as stomach trouble. Before using internally, I suggest taking the precautions mentioned above.

BERRY FRUITS such as Blue Berries have extremely good food qualities but also work well in regulating digestion, bladder infections, colds and sore throats. Elder Berry extract has recently been proven to be effective in the treatment of sore throat and flue symptoms. These are not powerful treatments but it's worth reviewing existing literature about these kinds of problems.

SAW PALMETTO BERRY extract in amounts of 300 mg or more per day are effective in the treatment of enlarged prostrate. I consider it to be more effective in combinations using vitamins and minerals good for prostate. However, saw palmetto berry seems to be the key product.

SPECIAL TEAS will be included in chapter 15 "Developing Your Own Treatment Plans." I mention three of these very special teas in closing this section because they are very helpful in many treatments. They are also used in preventative programs.

PAU D' ARCO is derived from the inner bark of a tree that grows in the Amazon region of South America. It is widely recognized as a blood cleanser and healing agent used by natives of the Amazon for hundreds of years. It can be purchased from health food stores in loose powder form or in capsules.

ESSIAC is an herbal remedy primarily used for treating and preventing cancer. It was originally developed in Canada by the Ojibwa Indians (before the time of the white man) and given to Rene Caisse after her treatment and recovery from cancer. The formula was reportedly given to nurse Caisse by an old medicine man. The ingredients can be individually purchased from herb shops that carry bulk herbs. The formula has been transferred to Elaine Alexander for marketing in the United under the name of Flor-Essence. I have seen products for sale under both names in the form of dried herbs ready for brewing, prepared tonics and capsuled extracts. This product will be given more detailed explanation in chapter 15.

GREEN TEA has been widely promoted in recent years as an excellent anti oxidant which promotes good health in a number of ways. It reportedly helps to prevent cancer and is used heavily in the orient as a health drink. It is recommended as a healthy substitute for coffee.

Read, study, experiment a little. What you know can not only save money and time, it may save your life. Think! And live a happy life.

Morris "J" Llewellyn

CHAPTER 12: ELECTRIC AND MAGNETIC

THERAPIES

This is an area of extremes. People have been jailed for not following established medical procedures, Quacks abound, miracles have happened, some areas of science (including medical science) have greatly advanced, and there is still plenty of controversy around.

Electric pulse machines, pulse machines used in connection with colored light applications to the various CHAKRAS supposedly hold the secrets to many miraculous healings. I have used a copy of the Rife Ray machine, examined the attendant literature and believe there is value and healing abilities involved. However, I find the whole thing too complicated for me but it may be worth knowing about. There is pertinent data available on the internet and in some reference books. This stuff is hard to understand and is very controversial.

There is another area of study that involves light and color which I have not incorporated into any of my own treatment plans. The doctor I know about who uses some of these techniques with reports of great success is William Campbell Douglas, MD. If you are interested in Light Therapy treatments or the many ways Photoluminescence is used in healing read his own book "Into the Light" for his research and treatment successes.

MAGNETIC THERAPIES are quite a different story. Use of magnetic treatments have been in use since before Cleopatra's lodestones. I don't see a real need for controversy about magnets in our time but we do have some. As I see it controversy about magnets comes from ignorance and failure to communicate.

I am upset to see some of the ignorance passed on to the public who have a right and a need to know the simple facts about magnets, especially when they are used for health and healing purposes. I am disappointed to see some of my favorite doctors selling health products aggressively and promoting magnetic products with no attendant information. Just to make some extra bucks. I don't mind the bucks for economic stimulation keeps us all going. It's the process that disturbs me. Cheap magnets are sold in great quantity in shoe liners, pain patches, and many products that impact health. No information is given, but it should be. Most of the products mentioned above are harmless if only used as promoted. However, the danger falls on people wanting to use magnets for serious ailments thinking they know something about magnetic treatments when they don't. They know a little but they need to know much more.

There are many strengths and configurations of magnets used in many useful applications. The message I want to convey here relates to magnets that are used in health applications. I have used magnets extensively in the treatment of my own cancer and other ailments. They do a great job. They do affect health at the cellular level in different ways.

PLEASE NOTE that if you intend to use magnets to treat a serious illness, make sure you consult with a health care professional who understands the many configurations of magnets and how to use them. For our purposes here I merely want to communicate what I know about magnetic products and some of the uses. This much information can help a lot when you talk to a practitioner about establishing a treatment plan involving magnets.

Polar orientation is very important in magnets used for health treatment. They are made to be bi-polar, positive pole or negative pole. Many industrial magnets and weaker magnets used in health care are not identified as to polar orientation or strength.

Strength and composition are the other major factors to be considered in magnets used for treatment. Strength, composition and polar orientation are all identifiable and measurable. Understanding these factors is essential for successful specific treatment applications.

I will summarize here the types of magnets I have in terms of material composition and strength:

CERAMIC SOLID STATE IRON OXIDE magnets I have measure in inches (2 x 5 x ½). Manufacturer lists strength at 4200 gauss. The flat plate of these ceramic magnets is placed over the infected area with the NORTH (negative) side facing the skin.

PLASTIFORM SOLID STATE IRON OXIDE magnets come in sheets 9 x 12 inches. These sheets can be cut to desired size and several thicknesses (to achieve desired strength) applied with non-allergenic tape enabling application to a variety of surfaces.

NEODYMIUM ALLOY magnets are circular disks (.3 thick x .8 inch diameter) are strong, effective and versatile. I used these disks extensively on my own cancer. I.e., they were an important part of my treatment program. Proper application is essential. One side North and one side South. Can be covered and applied with a good surgical, non-allergenic tape. Be certain of polar application always applying North side facing affected area.

There may be other configurations of magnets available but these have served me well. Always be certain of proper polar application. DO NOT TREAT TUMORS CANCEROUS CONDITIONS OR INFECTIONS

WITH SOUTH POLE FIELDS. USE NORTH FIELD for these conditions. I mark all my magnets with permanent marker to make sure I can always identify the correct polarization.

General consensus is that North pole energy has antibiotic properties (because it retards or controls infections). Conversely South pole has energy-giving properties. Therefore the North pole is most beneficial for pain and infections while the South Pole is helpful for pain from swellings, stimulating organ function, strengthening tissue and creating acidity.

According to Dr. Richard Broeringmeyer's research the following polar actions are indicated:

NORTH POLE ACTION:

1. Arrests protein activity

2. Draws Fluid

3. Contracts

4. Vaso-constricts

5. Increases Alkalinity

6. Acts to sedate and gives a calming effect

7. Inhibits and controls pain

8. Increases potassium ions

9. Decreases abnormal calcium ions

10. Increases mental alertness

11. Increases tissue oxygen

12. Slows multiplication of Micro-organisms

13. Fights infections

14. Attracts white & red blood cells to aid healing

15. Slows heart function

16. Decreases hydrogen & increases oxygen

SOUTH POLE ACTION:

1. Increases protein activity

2. Depresses fluid

3. Expands

4. Vaso-dilates

5. Enlarges

6. Increases acidity

7. Stimulates

8. Increases sodium

9. Speeds metabolic processes

10. Can irritate tissue

11. Can increase pain

12. Can increase heart beat and action

13. Speeds up multiplication of microorganisms

14. Decreases oxygenation of tissue

15. Increases hydrogen & decreases oxygen

I do not agree or disagree with every aspect of this research. The importance of this rather long list rests in the demonstration of the broad impact that magnetic application can have, and on the demonstrated differences in the effects of North (Negative) pole versus South (positive) pole.

What does all this mean to me personally? The scientific aspects of research of magnetic treatments should not be trivialized and the good results such as I have had should be authenticated and publicized. I also think this should apply to other areas of research about natural healing.

Morris "J" Llewellyn

CHAPTER 13: MIND CONTROL - VISUALIZATION

- SPIRITUAL HEALING

Of all the Natural Healing Efforts we have talked about and all of the wonderful advances of Modern American Medicine which we recognize, there is still one thing to consider. That is individual reality. We have many good cures, good treatments, and excellent techniques but these only serve to influences a condition. The brain and body must accept and apply such an influence to effect healing.

As near as I can tell the healing professions, including the medical profession, recognize the dimensions of human health as body, mind, and spirit. The medical people then go about concentrating on fixing the body. It is tangible, visible, and confined to the dimensions of the body. The body may be the simplest dimension to work with.

Medical researchers have done well pushing forward to the brink of known knowledge but seldom venture beyond the established dimension. Psychiatry has ventured ahead in some limited areas. This seems to me an indication of what we don't know.

I am troubled that individual reality has been completely left up to the individual. In an advanced technological society such as ours, much more help should be available for individuals stuck in this dimension.

As indicated earlier, I have developed my own treatment plans and have briefly ventured into elements of the healing process that are not well known. I am relating some of my own experiences categorized in areas and dimensions as I see them.

MIND CONTROL

MIND CONTROL for me is a special ability, acquired by continuous mental exercise. It gives me the ability, albeit somewhat limited, to calm and direct brain activity and establish control over pain and cellular function.

I have been working with mind control in one way or another for many years. To me, it has always meant what I could do with my mind or what I could get my mind to do with the rest of my body.

As a matter of curiosity I decided to look at the internet to see what other people had to say about mind control. I was surprised to see how little there was that paralleled anything I had done. There was a lot about elements of mind control such as visualization, various approaches to meditation, emotional control and counseling, and the mental effects of oriental and Ayurvedic (exercise) physical movement. It was good reading and I recommend it. What you know will be your greatest healing tool. For the purpose of my message to readers of this book, I will continue to relate my own healing experiences.

While on the internet and searching for parallels to my own activity, I found almost nothing under the name of Mind Control. While looking under that name, there were many thousands of reports listed under Mind Control. They all related to making victims of their subjects. Most of these reports were about research by secret military activities or by commercial efforts to promote products or ideas. It explained how some of this was done via our regular channels of communication. I.e., by television, radio, canned messages on telephones, the internet and even newspapers. Hell! I almost felt victimized just reading some of that stuff. What's my point by bringing this up here? This is not trivial data! It's even happening in ads about medicine. I bring it into this discussion here because we all need to recognize there is more than one kind of Mind Control. We need to be careful about what information we internalize. And, we need to exercise our own form of mind control. Think! And live a happy healthy life.

Probably the most well known form of mind control that relates to health is some form of meditation. Anyone can meditate. It merely means to reflect upon, study or ponder, to think deeply or continuously. It can mean to plan or ponder which is almost synonymous with contemplate.

Meditation has always been an important part of many religions. Its main purpose is to remove distractions from the mind. Hindu and Buddhist religions see it as a necessity to achieve spiritual enlightenment. Various things have been added to help avoid distraction or to direct focus such as breathing patterns. Transcendental meditation is a poplar method which includes sitting in a quiet room and using a mantra. The mantra usually takes the form of a chant and serves the purpose of avoiding distraction and directing focus.

Applied mind control has taken several forms and combinations in the United States. The popularity of these techniques developed in the 1960's and 1970's and has increased steadily because of many proven successes, even having edged into mainstream medicine. Mind control has been successfully applied in many areas of healing: Yoga Therapy, Relaxation Therapies, Visualization Therapies, Music Therapy, Meditation for stress relief, Energy Healing, Breath Healing and many applications of Biofeedback. When it comes to practical development and application these methods all seem to have meditation and relaxation as the base elements. The theories and applications are almost endless and would require several books to cover the subject. In holding to my own personal experiences, I must at least relate my experiences with visualization and spiritual healing.

VISUALIZATION

VISUALIZATION has been throughly introduced in recent years as useful for everything from relaxation to cancer treatment. It is only successful as a highly personalized program. Obviously the visualization must come from the person attempting to use the procedure. Begin the procedure as if you were to meditate. Assume a prone position on a bed or a recliner and avoid distraction both internal and external. At this point immerse your self into the visualization process rather than using a mantra.

As near as I can tell, my technique does not conflict with the basic principles I have read about. I have practiced my form of visualization since I learned it 12 years ago while developing my own cancer treatment program. I used recommendations I read about during my learning phase such as preparation of surroundings, invoking a relaxation response and using a mantra. I soon discovered that I could go through the preparation stages in a minute or two. I then went directly to the visualization.

In the beginning I had no idea how effective visualization could be. I was soon able to have an affect on organ activity, I could affect body chemistry and I could abate pain. Wow! After my first success I thought I had been endowed with some sort of special talent and was convinced that I had personal help from a Godly source.

I am a believer in the possibility of such things. However, I am certain such help is not required for successful visualization. As mentioned above, the first step is complete preparation as if getting ready for a serious session of meditation. Substitute a visualization for the traditional mantra. I do not believe in staging or practicing in the same sense as if learning a speech or preparing for an acting part in a play. Every time you attempt visualization, its for real. However. Practice does make perfect. Its possible to learn a bit of something new every time you do it.

How does one formulate a visualization? It is different for each person and each visualization. After all, we are each a complete and separate spiritual entity. Some people visualize improvements to their own personality such as being more relaxed, contentment, planning a lifetime event, etc. As for me, I have always formulated my visualization attempts around a health issue. To do this I have diagnostic data available if possible. If I do not have diagnostic information, I will begin working with symptoms. I identify the organs involved. I study the situation as much as possible and find out what kind of healing events I want to take place. The more facts you start with the better. My visualization becomes a directive or a request for the body to perform effectively in its effort to heal. This message to your own body effectively becomes your mantra. While working with it there is no other influence in your existence. Over a period of time, such as while working with cancer, it is necessary to use this procedure many times. It is a treatment. If it helps, keep using it, perhaps it will require a long time to effect a complete healing.

After using a visualization for a single purpose, repeating it often makes it easy. By concentrating on the message intently you become its only purpose and necessary changes come automatically. Just doing this is an amazing experience. You become good at it and you become able to perform other similar functions with ease.

SPIRITUAL HEALING

SPIRITUAL HEALING is an essential part of a complete healing. I have seen strange manifestations of spiritual healing. The source, the technique and the results seem to come in various ways within various cultures and by different shamans. I am convinced that the result is all that counts and that complete healing will escape the person who is not spiritually well.

The next few paragraphs will describe some of the sources of such healing.

People see "spiritual healing" in different ways such as making peace with oneself and with others or seeking some kind of connection with Deity. I am sure this is part of it. But there are many more avenues of spiritual healing. In my mind, I see a spiritual healing when someone can actually attest to feeling well because of an infusion of some kind of power.

About ten years ago, while I was treating my own cancer, I read an article about a New York woman who had been released from a local hospital as a hopeless case. She was high spirited and determined so she went to a Japanese hospital willing to take "last resort" cases. This hospital also gave her no hope. As a last resort she flew to a New Guinea hospital known to be staffed by local shamans. As the story goes she was admitted. Shortly thereafter her doctor arrived. He was a local "witch doctor." His tools consisted of an herbal concoction (immediately administered), colorful headdress and staff, a smoke pot and a large feather. His treatment consisted of dance and incantations. The entire routine was rhythmic, loud and smokey. It lasted until shortly after dawn. At which time he ended with a short routine that consisted of passing the feather from head to foot. As the story was told, she arose and went home supposedly cured. As I recall, the source was one of the national weekly papers. Perhaps not a very reliable source.

This story of spiritual healing is the most far-out I have encountered because of the setting. For the sake of demonstrating a point, lets say it is completely true. Did the healing come from the power of the shaman? His calls for help from his God? The herbal medication? The affect of the music? The rhythmic beat? Or the healing power initiated within her own brain?

This story is not as crazy as it sounds. Each of the possibilities listed can be demonstrated as existing in our own culture:

Calling upon the Spirit is very common in our culture and it has been done since the creation. I have seen spiritual healing realized through prayer by individuals, prayer by religious authority and by systematic routines such as energy transfer and combinations of faith, prayer, energy transfer and Devine intervention. Most of us have heard of miraculous healing within our own religions. The validity of healing by prayer has been proven by surveys at hospitals showing those who are prayed for realize more healing than those who are not prayed for. An interesting development in recent years is how many hospitals now allow religious involvement and some actually request what is known as "Touch Therapy" to be a part of the recovery process.

If you want verification study scientific reports of prayer and energy transfer. Also read up on Reiki, an ancient healing art, practiced by Tibetan healers for over a thousand years.

Reiki was introduced to the modern world by the Japanese in the 19th century. In Japanese Reiki means "universal life force."

It is practiced by trained practitioners. The object is to revitalize body, mind, and spirit by calling upon the universal life energy. Theoretically, this technique is easy to learn and can be practiced by oneself.

I have never used a practitioner of Reiki. However, I have observed, and used, free lance operators that use energy transfer in a variety of ways. I have trained myself to use energy in applied kinesiology. I can effectively muscle test to identify various sensitivities. I am not really good at energy transfer or testing because I don't do it much anymore. I do know the skill is easy to acquire and I know the process is valid and it can be very effective.

I don't mean to lay it on that poor old Shaman "witch doctor" but whether he knew it or not, he was applying some very valid concepts. I am referring to the healing benefits of music and rhythmic beat which have been a part of every culture since the beginning. And perhaps the most relied on in ancient times, Spiritual Healing. These elements have always been a part of every healing ritual. We still have the vestiges of some ancient rituals in modern healing.

I was fortunate enough to see and experience a phase of musical and rhythmic projection from the past into the future. At the time I saw this happening, I was impressed and fascinated but mostly entertained.

I lived in Brazil five years (1953 - 1958). At least three years were spent in Salvador, Bahia, Brazil which is known as the center of the Afro-Brazilian religions, most prominently represented by Candomble.

Back then I had no interest in the healing arts as such. But there was no way could I have escaped seeing what I saw nor could I have totally avoided involvement. I lived on the brink of a hill in the city of Salvador. Almost every Saturday night the rhythmic roll of drums could be heard coming from neighborhoods below. The drums of Candomble were a part of religious ceremonies brought to Brazil by African slaves. Their descendants now make up a large part of the Salvador Bahia's population and Candomble is more prevalent than ever. These ceremonies permeate the religious, spiritual and health lives of a large segment of the local population. I had domestic employees and many acquaintances who were African Brazilian. Many of them relied on these ceremonies for social and healing guidance. I have been a guest at several of these ceremonies and tried to observe what really happens. It is impossible to take it all in. There is a person who guides the proceedings (a chanter) and demonstrates some authority. The total program consists of stories, singing, and music. The theme is dominated by drums which roll out a rhythmic chant. Many people go into a convulsive like state, see visions, and proclaim healing. It was obvious that some people remained in an altered state for several days.

Obviously these people, whatever they are, healers, entertainers or spiritual channels, operate in an atmosphere of isolation, healing, hypnotizing, and influencing. The condition of isolation comes from geographic confinement, their very unique experience and a low level of formal education. I mention this because it is one of the examples of techniques that still exist and are practiced by millions of people. Valid healing methods are involved.

These healing arts are not frivolous games but are the remains of religions brought to this part of the world by the Brazilian slave trade. Most of the arrivals came from the Congo, Angola, and Mozambique around 1570.

Its too bad we cannot benefit more from this isolated culture. Its also too bad that we also suffer from a type of isolation, much different than theirs of course. In our culture, if healing is involved, if it can't be patented, if it isn't a drug, and if it doesn't turn a handsome profit, don't bother!

Thank goodness we live in a democracy. If we don't break the law, we can still set our own course. Just be careful in the area of health treatments. Special interests have been able to pass many laws that favor their position and discriminate against any competition.

We are fortunate to have many among us who are determined to do good. They love truth and they love people. Consequently we can benefit from knowing the past and being able to perpetuate truth. This seems to be working well in spiritual healing and in music. I need to say a bit more about the effects of music in our own culture.

I used classical music as a companion to meditation in my own cancer treatment program. I knew what I liked to hear, and it was very soothing. I really didn't need to know much about the mechanics or the history of music.

I was, however, very pleased when I learned that Music therapy and sound healing therapies are now recognized and therapists are board certified. For me, music can be very stimulating, soothing, or comforting by merely tuning into the appropriate selection.

In Greek mythology, Apollo was the God of music as well as the God of medicine. At various places in the scriptures music is used to sooth the soul. Today music therapy programs have been established in several American universities. And in 1950, the National Association for Music Therapy was established. These few facts highlight the importance of music in our culture for both mental and physical healing.

So what! How can I tell if a certain kind of music will help me with my stress related illness or with mood disorders, or just with my general health? Since we are all different, it is not appropriate to create a general musical menu. However, a good ground rule is to pick your preference of something you perceive as soft, soothing, pleasant, and interesting. That method surely works for me.

While looking for suggestions relative to this same problem, a music therapist suggested formulating your own list of favorites within each of the following catagories:

Classical - such as:

Bach-"Air for the G-String"

Beethoven-"Moonlight Sonata", "Pastoral Symphony"

Brahms-"Lullaby"

Chopin-"Nocturne in G"

Debussy-"Clair de Lune"

Handel-"Water Music"

Saint-Saens-"The Swan"

Schubert-"Ave Maria"

Vivaldi-"The Four Seasons"

Classical is highly recommended because it is complex and moving. But make your own choice. Be sure to add your own selections to the following catagories:

Symphonic

Piano

Guitar

Country

Sound tracks - recommended: "Born Free", Chariots of Fire", and "The Sound of Music".

There is no doubt that music constitutes an important part of Spiritual Healing. It has been called the Language of the Soul.

Use it with pleasure in successful healing.

Morris "J" Llewellyn

CHAPTER 14: DEVELOPING YOUR OWN

TREATMENT PLAN

The key to developing your own treatment plan is to make sure it is your own. It can't come from me, some health food store expert, or even a doctor. Even though such people can be very helpful, you need to know your own plan and what you are trying to do with it. I make a few changes to my plan from time to time. I make changes because my needs change and my knowledge of products slowly expands. I consult with several sympathetic doctors from time to time about my natural treatments and my ailments.

Just a note about doctors. They need to be sympathetic toward you and your unique situation. I have several good ones. There are usually some good ones around. The reason I bring this subject up several times is that it is dangerous to not know who and what you are dealing with. I could never completely surrender myself to the care of anyone. However, I have surrendered myself on various occasions to receive specific surgeries or medical services that I understand from a doctor that understands me.

So, with that said, we can concentrate on the best way for anyone to establish their own treatment plan, for almost anything.

First, develop a plan that is uniquely yours starting with the basics. If you have any questions about basics review chapters 9 and 10.

A basic plan will, of course, start with your choice of a basic supplement package of vitamins and minerals. As you will see in the following comments, many things can be added to a basic program in an effort to care for specific ailments. I have added many individual products for that reason. Be cautious not to add additional combinations without careful study. The thing to be avoided in adding combinations is the progressive accumulation of some ingredients you may not want in large quantities.

Secondly, your basic plan will include additional items chosen to assist with any specific problem you may want to treat. By adding two or three books, we could cover most of the possibilities. But, I have a much easier way. Even though your plan must be unique and may be developed with assistance such as mentioned in earlier chapters, I will give some examples that may be used as guidelines. I.e., I will detail the specific protocols I have used for the disorders listed below:

CANCER - When treating my lymphoma (a cleaved small cell lymphoma) many people came to me for advice. Obviously, I can not give what equates to medical advice, nor diagnose nor treat illness. And I have never done so. I can only say what I did for myself and what I think the reaction was within my own body. And, possibly what my view is of some available products and treatments.

It is good to start with a standard medical diagnosis if possible. It is good to know what you are dealing with. What would I do about:

Taking Chemotherapy - For me, no. However, after good consultation I would consider it for lymphomas and some leukemia. My personal view was I could do better with energy transfer and tonics. This was discussed in chapters 11 and 12.

Radiation - For me, probably never! My personal substitution for radiation was effective use of magnets.

Attitude - is very important - Be fearless, positive, and in good cheer. Also follow previous suggestions on mind control, visualization, meditation, and prayer. These things can equate to some of the best medicine there is. Life style is also a determinate of every aspect of health.

Now that the base line supplementation has been determined and the life style established to stimulate maximum effectiveness, there are specific foods, tonics, and natural herbs that can do wonders for some people. Remember, these things are in addition to the base line treatment. For a helpful diet, reduce animal products, increase vegetables, grain products should come from grain that is not milled or processed. Eliminate sweets, limit artificial sweeteners unless you are diabetic. Eliminate soda pop - substitute strong caffeinated drinks with green tea. Green tea has its own healing properties.

The following products can be added to a cancer treatment program. When added individually follow usage instructions on the container. They can be added over time as needed. This period of time can be as much as a few years. My own program was intense for about two years and tapered down over the past ten years. I mention this time factor because you will change some things over time. However it is appropriate to never completely end a routine of good health. Even if many items can be eliminated from the program, the basic supplementation should go on indefinitely. This also applies to life style improvements and exercise. The basic program will usually have plenty of the required vitamins and minerals. The exception is vitamin C and the minerals potassium, calcium, and magnesium which are needed in larger quantities for some serious illnesses.

The tonic Essiac (Also known as flor-essence) is extremely good for cancer and it is adaptogenic for other ailments. Pau D'Arco (the inner bark of a tree from the Amazon) is usually made into a tea but is also available in capsules. It is used widely to treat cancer and infections.

Laetrile has been very controversial as a cancer treatment since it was promoted as a cure without convincing proof by alternative doctors in the U.S. and Mexico several years ago. It may be worth a try. I used it as an adjunct treatment in my program. A safe and easy way to get it is taking bitter apricot pits, available at any health food store.

CANDIDA ALBICANS (yeast overgrowth) and other intestinal imbalances can be terribly disabling and troublesome.

After many exploratory treatments for cancer which included a number of antibiotics, I became burdened by terrific intestinal problems. One of the symptoms was at least a year of diarrhea. I was (as always) using my basic supplement program which did not help this problem. I consulted with medical doctors and used a number of their recommendations. Nystatin powder was helpful, but it really didn't do the job.

I make it a point to study some of the many reports I get and was impressed by the reports published by LIFESTAR International, Inc., Advanced Nutritional Systems, San Francisco, California 94103, USA. I ordered their probiotic for personal use called (ProTec).

I began taking this product according to label instructions and experienced dramatic elimination of digestive problems within ten days.

This is the best example I have of how "medicine" can't always cure a problem, but may actually cause it. Since that time I have used recommended amounts of probiotics and digestive enzymes and have had no digestive problems. There are several good sources for similar products. Some of them are at your local health food store.

Even though GERD is an ailment involving the upper parts of the intestinal tract, it responds to similar treatments using probiotics and digestive enzymes. The so called "heartburn" is distressing and painful when extreme. And when left untreated for a long period of time, it can be dangerous. Some very short term relief is available from a variety antacids, both off the shelf and by prescription. A note of caution - too much use of anti acids, especially prescription drugs that stop acid production can cause damage to the normal digestive functions with disastrous results. For some daily treatments see my **MEDICINE CABINET** listed below.

DIABETES - I don't know a great deal about this disorder but feel compelled to mention a few things about it. This disorder is DEADLY and should not be ignored. Why do I think this is one of the most deadly diseases? Because it aggravates any other disorders that may exist in the body. Even a scratch is harder to heal if one is diabetic!

A rather complicated condition of imbalanced cellular chemistry is involved. If you are diabetic you should have a medical doctor who is specialized in this complicated disorder. Especially if you have Type I diabetes. Type II is much more responsive to natural treatments but you should still work with a doctor. Have an glycosylated hemoglobin (HbA1c)test every three months which is a test indicating blood sugar control for the preceding three months.

There are many natural healing items that can be helpful. Chromium is a natural regulator of metabolism. I prefer to use Chromium Picolinate which is a well tolerated form of chromium. If one is diabetic, sugar and lack of exercise raises hell with the entire system! That's something we can all do a lot about. Why don't we? I would say it is too much TV and weak will power.

The following natural products are also useful in treating type II diabetes. I use several of these and merely follow label instructions. Vanadium is a trace mineral, Biotin is a vitamin B, Niacin is recommended as an aid to carbohydrate metabolism, and Magnesium is thought to aid the effects of insulin in the cells. Fenugreek is a popular spice in some eastern countries. It reportedly regulates glucose metabolism. It is available in health food stores as a spice, in combinations, and as a tea. There are also other herbals that are recommended by Ayurvedic, Indian, and Chinese. I have not evaluated their use in my own program. All these things may be worth discussing with your special doctor. This disorder is so elusive and dangerous that whatever you do should be discussed with him.

MY MEDICINE CABINET - Incorporates two kinds of treatments:

A few serious treatments that are important as an independent treatment, and could also be an essential element in the treatment of serious disease.

Or, the other kind, herbs, tonics or "off the shelf" items that I use all the time for various ailments. These things may help cancer but they do wonders when secondary problems come along such as colds, allergies, stomach upsets, or minor injuries.

On the heavy side, the most important item in my medicine cabinet is a **detoxification process**. There are times when everyone needs to be detoxified. If you are a young, energetic, dissipating and self abusing person and you think you are related to superman and doubt the coming of your day of reckoning, you are having a pipedream that will turn into a nightmare. Most people will realize variations of this scenario. For most of us it is the unceremonious burning of youth and the reluctant welcoming of aging. Caution! There are a lot of pill salesmen out there selling supplements that "detoxify". This is only a small part of the picture.

Your body is made to detoxify itself, more pills may add to the already established overload. Our bodies were made to detoxify by working physically, sweating, getting sun and fresh air, being hungry part of the time and eating natural foods that are highly nutritious, getting appropriate rest and having efficient evacuation of body wastes. How does one do all that! Well, we need help at times.

We have all studied, or at least been informed, about exercise, diet, and supplementation. Even if conscientious, some of us can have a lot of trouble with toxicity. Its easy to spot in yourself, as well as others. Look for excess fat, fatigue, mental fog, poor elimination of body waste, and a variety of skin problems. What's the cure? Its easy to identify. Much harder to administer. I have been there a few times myself. My Medicine Cabinet has some of the answers:

1.   Practice the principles of diet, supplementation and exercise explained in this book and many other places.

2.   Take a detoxifying hot bath two times a week. Add the following to the water: 2 cups of sea salt or rock salt, 2 cups of soda and two cups of cider vinegar. I like to use a jet tub for this one. It is relaxing and feels good.

3.   Use a dry Sauna twice weekly on days the hot bath is not used. Be sure to use the safety precautions that come with the Sauna equipment. Don't overdo it.

4.   A less heard of practice that is very effective even with cancer and other serious health problems is intestinal cleansing. This is not

effectively done with drugs. The very best and most reliable means is colonic wash and high enemas. I have used a nurse trained in doing colonic cleansing for a short time when I was very ill.

Almost as effective, however, is a high enema routine which I developed. It calls for using 1 & 1/2 to 2 quarts of warm clean water. Add garlic powder from 6 capsules containing 500 mg each. Repeat two or three times per week. Any pure garlic powder should work. I use Garolic - 500 mg per capsule from DNA Labs, Chelan, WA 98816. This is much better than the coffee enema recommended by some health plans. Garlic is a natural healing agent and is beneficial to the body in many ways. Whereas, coffee is a strong drink that is harmful to the body as a whole.

On the lighter side, my **MEDICINE CABINET** contains many items. I use some of these items every day and others I use infrequently for emergencies. I also use this part of my medicine cabinet as a part of my ongoing study and experimentation. I recommend this for everyone because we are all different. It is good to learn more about oneself. Warning! Be careful. Don't use dangerous drugs without proper guidance. And keep it legal.

I am closing this chapter with a list of some of the remaining items in my Medicine cabinet and what I use them for. I hope it will be useful to readers as a guideline for useful products. Your list will eventually be much better for you than mine could ever be.

CAYENNE PEPPER is the most used product in my medicine cabinet. I use it every day. I have used it in such great quantities that I make my own extract from powdered cayenne and pure grain alcohol.

My personal use of cayenne is for stimulating heart function and circulation. I also use it for stomach problems such as ulcers. It has been very effective for me in these areas for many years. I have used it as a post heart attack tonic in place of nitroglycerin. It worked well for me.

Cayenne appears in many ointments and salves used for pain control and skin disorders. The best examples are arthritis pain and shingles treatment.

I recommend that all herbs be purchased ready to use from an herb shop that carries a full line of herbal products. Dr. Christopher's original herbal formulas, Springville, Utah 84663, 1-800-453-1406 is a reliable source. They carry dried herbs in the original form as well as prepared powders and extracts.

Cayenne can be used in a variety of forms and strengths. Many variations of the hot red pepper family are used around the world. It is very commonly used in some Asian countries as a vegetable and a staple food. According to the studies I have read there is very little cardiovascular and intestinal illness among people who use a lot of cayenne as a part of their diet.

The rest of the **items in my medicine cabinet** are listed in no particular order. Each item listed is effective for the given purpose and becomes very important when needed.

Colloidal silver is a natural antibiotic. It can be used internally or externally and comes in various forms and strengths.

I have used the liquid for rashes, skin growths, and minor injuries. I have found 10 ppm very effective for eye irritations (such as pink eye) and sinus infections. Use in the same manner as nose drops. The ointment (uses 40 ppm or greater) is a mix of colloidal silver and aloe vera which **I use** for many skin disorders, minor burns, and as an underarm deodorant.

BLUE STAR OINTMENT is a terrific healing treatment for pain and itching caused by ring worm, athletes foot, jock itch, and minor injuries. The only active ingredient is CAMPHOR. I was only recently acquainted with this product but I am impressed with its usefulness. It is available off the shelf at most drug stores.

HYDROGEN PEROXIDE is a very useful treatment for many things such as gargles, mouth wash, and as a cleansing disinfectant. Many uses and instructions for such uses are given on the label. Naturopathic doctors often use this item as a treatment for serious illness. Consult with such a doctor before using in this manner. One of the great things about this product is the low cost and abundant availability at any pharmacy or grocery store.

POTENCE AND HEALTHY PROSTRATE PRODUCTS: Of course there are many products readily available in any health food store - some good, some not so good. I mention some of the products I keep in my **MEDICINE CABINET** because there are several uses for some of these products. Some of these items are essential for older men. If you plan on self medicating, do so with some professional advice.

If you use these products in combination, be sure you are familiar with the ingredients and don't let the combination become too complicated.

There are many products on the market that claim remarkable results when used for impotence. Be careful! Avoid most of it. At the older ages, especially over 65, most men need to give special attention to the care of the prostate gland. And many also need to treat impotence. Many of the products that advertise certain relief for both problems don't work very well. My view on this is that the two problems should be treated separately even though they may be related. If you are not absolutely sure of what you are doing, get some advise from a Urologist that is willing to use natural products. These ailments can be a bit complicated and trying every product that comes along is expensive and sometimes dangerous.

My view is that the prostate should be treated first with a good product that contains a daily dosage of at least:

320 mg - Saw Palmetto Berries 4:1 extract

100 mg - Pygeum Africanum Bark 30:1 extract

200 mg - Pumpkin Seed 4:1 extract

100 mg - Urtica Dioica - Nettle Leaf Powder

100 mg - Swedish Flower Pollen Extract

20 mg - Lycopene Complex

---

800 I.U. - Vitamin D-3

30 mg - Zinc

100 mcg - Selenium

1.0 mg - Copper

These are the essential products in the supplement I use. A few "additional" vitamins and minerals appear in some other good products.

After using a good prostate supplement for a month, if any problem remains, you may need hormone supplementation. In this area, I use only natural products prepared by a compounding pharmacist, which are prescribed by my favorite doctor. Testosterone and/or DHEA are commonly needed.

I want to mention one additional item in this area that can be very useful for urinary/bladder problems. Cranberries. They can be used in several ways as juices, compotes, and extracts. I like the foods but my favorite when using for healing is the convenience of encapsulated dry extracts.

LECITHIN is an amazing product that provides a special form of nutrition we often miss, **Phosphatidyl Choline.** This product is often very helpful for nervous problems. When combined with vitamin B complex, especially B-12, dramatic improvement can sometimes be realized by people with a deficiency. I use it as a nerve toning tonic.

ORGANIC FLAX SEED OIL is an essential oil most of us should probably be using, given the nature of our modern diet. Flax seed is one of nature's richest and purest sources of the essential fatty acid Omega three (linolenic acid). I take it as a means of enriching my diet.

CLA (CONJUGATED LINOLEIC ACID) is another product I take to improve my diet. I use TONALIN XS-CLA, a product of Natures Way. It's purpose is to help reduce body fat and increase muscle tone. CLA used to be provided naturally with the use of beef and diary products. Current methods of feeding and caring for cattle have decreased CLA at its natural source.

DIGEST EASE is a dietary product (available from Natures Distributors, Fountain Hills. AZ 85268 - 1-800-624-7114) that provides probiotics, digestive enzymes and homeopathic enzymes. I have found it to be very helpful in establishing and maintaining bacterial balance throughout the intestinal tract. I use this product as an agent for balancing bacteria and recommend such a product for everyone. A similar product was identified above as an element of my very serious treatment for Candida Albicans. These products vary in stability but, in my opinion, they are essential for a good diet in today's drug oriented health care environment. Read the literature and ask for information. There is a lot of it available.

RHEUMATOID ARTHRITIS TREATMENTS: Rheumatoid Arthritis treatments can be very simple and effective. That is why I am listing together the effective ones I have used here with off-the-shelf stuff.

In my body, Arthritis may not be curable but I have been able to control it with ease. In the beginning I had to find the products that worked for me. That wasn't easy and it took some time. But since that time I have been astounded by what goes on. Many people are very sick with dangerous drugs used for treatment. If this were happening to me, I would insist on good results. Sadly in this world, I had to figure it out for myself. The following are the products that worked for me. I did have to determine which ones were best and how much to take. Label information helps a lot.

Glucosamine Sulfate with Condroitin and Vitamin C and Manganese in combination. I also incorporate Collagen (either Chicken

or beef - I prefer chicken). **MSM with extra minerals Potassium, Calcium, and Magnesium and extra Vitamins A,E, and C.**

The following **natural antibiotics: Olive Leaf Extract, Garlic. and Ginger can work wonders when bacterial infection and virus are involved as a cause of arthritis, and they were in my case.**

COMMON COLDS, FLUE, AND EMERGENCY TREATMENTS constitute most of the remaining items in my medicine cabinet. Most doctors settle for fluids, a light diet, and a weeks rest for treatment of a **COMMON COLD.** Of course, we must throw in all the new stuff being put out by pharmaceutical companies. Most of it is profitable for someone but doubtful as a cure. That is my opinion of course. My self treatment for a cold usually gives good results in two days or less, especially if treatment begins at first sign of symptoms. I.e., extra **fluids, colloidal silver as nose drops, two grams or more of vitamin C daily during duration of cold, licorice extract for throat, extra zinc, Vicks Vapor rub for comfort, Echinacea Augustifolia per label instruction if cold is persistent.** If flue develops add **Elderberry extract.** If flue is accompanied by a high temperature, I call the doctor immediately. I get good results with this routine. Sometimes the nose drops are all that is required.

For **EMERGENCY BELLY ACHE** which is usually caused by overeating and gas, I use a product called **GAS EASE.** It is a combination of **Cayenne, Papin, Slippery Elm Bark, Caraway seed, Ginger root, and Catnip herb.** This is the best product in my medicine cabinet for quick easy relief. This is an easy one and I mention it as an example of some of the good things that can end up in your medicine cabinet. Good, safe, things that are inexpensive and useful. Over the years I have acquired a small group of things I consider my own.

A good medicine cabinet is a great thing to have. It serves most of my health problems very well, there have been many. One last recommendation that is often overlooked by doctors and by people who treat themselves, the use of essential oils and homeopathic medicines. I use a few of these products with pleasure and success but the field of information is so large that I can only recommend looking into it. There is a lot of good stuff available from health food stores and Homeopathic Healers.

I wish all those people who want to be in charge of their own health, **GOOD LUCK AND GOOD HEALTH!**

CHAPTER 15: ADJUSTMENTS

After having lived with this extremely flawed immune system for seventy five years, I have learned a lot by merely surviving. I think the most important thing I have learned that will assure good physical and mental health is the importance of making proper adjustments.

As we grow and mature, we make appropriate adjustments automatically. By the age of six we start to adjust to not depending on Mother for food and total care. By eight we start to learn independence and righteous behavior and continue to grow and adjust accordingly.

We are all acutely aware of, and look forward to, the age milestones of 16, 18, and 21. These ages are times of important adjustments involving maturity, education, and progression to appropriate levels of legal responsibility.

As we go beyond these levels that are predefined, we all set our own individual course, have various levels of success, and encounter a variety of obstacles that may change our planned course.

Sometimes? No, most of the times when we experience a major obstacle or a course changing event, it will impact physical, psychological, and social aspects of our lives, including health factors. To remain useful, productive and healthy citizens, we must make appropriate adjustments that preserve our happiness and sense of self worth.

I hate most "shrink" work and I am not adequate to write a long chapter on making happy lives out of problems. So, with the reader's indulgence, I am going to relate three examples of life changing events from my own life. Hopefully, it will be easy to see what I am driving at when you read about these events.

EVENT ONE. Prior to college, my life was eventful and interesting with my share of problems. But for purposes of this example I will begin with college graduation.

I graduated with a degree in Political Science and a minor in Russian language. I did graduate work in International Law and Trade. As yet I was not fully prepared to seek the career I had hoped for as a top Political Officer assigned to Treaty Negotiation. Consequently, I accepted a lower administrative position with the State Department, Foreign Service. I adjusted to this with the goal of advancing to a better paying job in the Service. I liked my work. I seemed to be made for that kind of life. I loved living abroad and learning new languages like Greek and Portuguese. I was now married and had a child. After ten years, I decided the future was not lucrative enough and made the difficult decision to resign. According to my seniors, ten years of specialized activity in government made me worthless to any other activity. I had to prove them wrong.

I resigned from the Foreign Service, went to California unprepared for anything else, obtained a beginning position as a management trainee with a large aerospace firm.

This entailed drastic social changes, some assignments I didn't like and the beginning of health problems mentioned in the earlier parts of this book. How did I handle this situation?

First of all, I did not try to discard or forget my previous years of cherished and interesting experiences. It was an interesting chapter in my life which I still value very much. I looked at this new chapter as an opportunity to have new experiences. It was as if I had the opportunity for a new life. In a way that was true. Anyway, at this point, I didn't have much choice. This was not a defeat, it was a new opportunity and I took it to the limits of my ability. I worked in that industry for 25 years. Over time I received several awards and many rewards of higher pay and better assignments. I had to self educate myself as part of this process and today I look upon that experience as an interesting and exciting career from which I am now retired.

The point I am making here is that appropriate adjustments are sometimes necessary. Doing what is necessary and doing it well can be very rewarding to mental and physical health.

EVENT TWO. Most adjustments are not as complex as the one depicted in event one. Event two required an adjustment more common in middle age. It is simple to identify, and strictly health related, but if the adjustment is not made it can destroy the victim's life.

I was 45 years old, very energetic and still looking for more money and more satisfaction. However, I was committed to side activities that used up most of my extra time and energy. I still enjoyed the vices of the Foreign Service such as moderate drinking, heavy smoking, and a busy social life.

I was in an important meeting one morning with some policy making executives. Suddenly, I felt strange and very ill. I excused myself, left the room suddenly, and walked directly to the medical department. I arrived just in time to collapse into the lap of a strong lady nurse. I was having a heart attack. That was the beginning of a new phase in my life. Suddenly, life style adjustments were necessary.

I was now confined to the number one job, my family, and a new set of health rules. At a point like this one can be very much afraid, depressed and self pitying.

It is important not to buy into that scene. There is always a positive side to any situation. You must find it and act upon it. I was prayerfully thankful that I had a good recovery considering the seriousness of the situation.

Giving up the weed was very difficult but it was a strengthening experience. I gave it up "cold turkey" and suffered the process for almost a year but I still benefit from the experience. As a result, I am much healthier physically and my mental state was greatly improved. I learned to benefit from a determined attitude and improved confidence. My life was improved in the long term.

If one doesn't look for these positive elements, they can be missed, and missing the positive side can be very detrimental.

EVENT THREE. The third event was when I received the diagnosis of cancer and given a prognosis of less than six months to live. I was expected to submit to the painful process of chemotherapy and radiation which I would not accept. The entire experience was related in chapters five and seven.

My confidence and determination had already been fortified by previous experiences but my self treatment and ultimate cure were in a sense my ultimate victory and crowning glory. I could have been swayed to another direction by some of the following rationale.

After a painful exploratory surgery and the disappointing diagnosis, I could have accepted this period as a good time to die. After all, I had no dependant children, I did not want to be a burden on anyone, by dying I could avoid a lot of pain and difficulty, and I could have passed on comfortably causing little or no inconvenience to anyone. Anyway, maybe it was the right time for me. I was in my mid-sixties and had done well to reach that age.

My innermost self had been conditioned to fight and strive and I now know there is joy and satisfaction in exercising this attitude. If I could give a message to anyone having similar experiences it would be this.

"Do your best to live as long and as good as you can. You will never know the joy and excitement of new experiences and expanded knowledge if you don't take the trip. If you pray and beg for life and happiness you may be rewarded. But, you can be sure when it is your time, He will come and take you in an instant and you can not stop it." So I say, give it your very best and enjoy the rewards.

The last twelve years of my life have been full of adjustments. I have made them as best as I could and moved forward with confidence. All the education and experiences of my earlier life have been wonderful. However, they didn't come close to equaling the rewards of the last twelve years. What were the rewards? Understanding, insights, a growing family, the excitement of learning new things that didn't exist in my earlier life. And, the anticipation of receiving more of the same.

Morris "J" Llewellyn

ABOUT THE AUTHOR

The introduction to this book is essential to the reader being able to understand my purpose, my intense interest in health issues, and the reasons why this book was written.

I was born in a small Utah town in 1927. These were difficult years of the great depression. Doctors, midwives, and other health practitioners of the times were very willing to travel in open country making house calls. It was common back then for health practitioners to vary greatly in their skills and backgrounds. From that time to this I have had an interest in how healing takes place and what roles are played by the patient, the health practitioner, and the unknown forces of the universe. I still see a significant influence by all of these elements in the healing process.

The advancement of science has (in my mind) only increased the evidence that there are many influences in the healing process and that today we are faced with an even greater body of the unknown. Each time we discover a new dimension of understanding we open up a vast universe of unknowns. The work in genetic research and DNA exemplifies this principle.

This book is a partial personal history which reveals a great deal of information about health practices. It reflects what I have learned about staying healthy, getting sick, reversing the disease process and regaining good health.

This book is not intended to be a technical reference.

In the medical field doctors and patients are both victimized. Pressures for greater profits are probably the number one cause. A stream of new medicines improperly introduced into medical practice are overwhelming doctors and endangering patients. Efforts external to medical practice are injected into the system which endanger patients and breakdown the doctor/patient relationship. One of the main problems is the extensive use of HMO's.

Yesterdays science has become today's lie. Profit opportunities bury truth for the purpose of perpetuating profit

The world is in political, social, religious, economic, and scientific turmoil. What is true? What is false? Much of the time it is hard to tell. This book only deals with the health care issue. I have tried to relate what I have done on my own. I hope I have shed some light on what we all can do about these issues. I implore you to exercise your rights and do what you can for yourself. If you do, it will ultimately benefit us all.

www.ingramcontent.com/pod-product-compliance
Lightning Source LLC
Chambersburg PA
CBHW031123180526
45160CB00001B/9